Hematologic Diseases

Editors

MAUREEN OKAM ACHEBE
ARIC PARNES

PRIMARY CARE: CLINICS IN OFFICE PRACTICE

www.primarycare.theclinics.com

Consulting Editor
JOEL J. HEIDELBAUGH

December 2016 • Volume 43 • Number 4

ELSEVIER

1600 John F. Kennedy Boulevard • Suite 1800 • Philadelphia, Pennsylvania, 19103-2899

http://www.theclinics.com

PRIMARY CARE: CLINICS IN OFFICE PRACTICE Volume 43, Number 4
December 2016 ISSN 0095-4543, ISBN-13: 978-0-323-47749-9

Editor: Jessica McCool
Developmental Editor: Colleen Viola

Primary Care: Clinics in Office Practice (ISSN: 0095–4543) is published quarterly by Elsevier Inc., 360 Park Avenue South, New York, NY 10010-1710. Months of issue are March, June, September, and December. Periodicals postage paid at New York, NY and additional mailing offices. Subscription prices are $225.00 per year (US individuals), $434.00 (US institutions), $100.00 (US students), $275.00 (Canadian individuals), $491.00 (Canadian institutions), $175.00 (Canadian students), $345.00 (international individuals), $491.00 (international institutions), and $175.00 (international students). Foreign air speed delivery is included in all *Clinics* subscription prices. All prices are subject to change without notice. POSTMASTER: Send address changes to *Primary Care: Clinics in Office Practice*, Elsevier Periodicals Customer Service, 11830 Westline Industrial Drive, St. Louis, MO 63146. Customer Service Health Sciences Division, Subscription Customer Service, 3251 Riverport Lane, Maryland Heights, MO 63043. **Customer Service: 1-800-654-2452 (U.S. and Canada); 314-447-8871 (outside U.S. and Canada). Fax: 314-447-8029. E-mail: journalscustomerservice-usa@elsevier.com (for print support); journalsonlinesupport-usa@elsevier.com (for online support).**

Reprints. For copies of 100 or more, of articles in this publication, please contact the Commercial Reprints Department, Elsevier Inc., 360 Park Avenue South, New York, NY 10010-1710. Tel. 212-633-3874; Fax: 212-633-3820; E-mail: reprints@elsevier.com.

Primary Care: Clinics in Office Practice is covered in *MEDLINE/PubMed (Index Medicus)* and *EMBASE/ Excerpta Medica, Current Contents/Clinical Medicine, and ISI/BIOMED.*

Contributors

CONSULTING EDITOR

JOEL J. HEIDELBAUGH, MD, FAAFP, FACG
Clinical Professor, Departments of Family Medicine and Urology; Clerkship Director, Department of Family Medicine, University of Michigan Medical School, Ann Arbor, Michigan; Ypsilanti Health Center, Ypsilanti, Michigan

EDITORS

MAUREEN OKAM ACHEBE, MD, MPH
Division of Hematology, Brigham and Women's Hospital; Hematology Services, Dana-Farber Cancer Institute, Assistant Professor, Harvard Medical School, Boston, Massachusetts

ARIC PARNES, MD
Instructor, Division of Hematology, Brigham and Women's Hospital; Dana-Farber Cancer Institute, Boston, Massachusetts

AUTHORS

JUNAID ARSHAD, MD
St. Mary's Hospital, Waterbury, Connecticut

JOHN ASTLE, MD, PhD
Department of Pathology, Yale University School of Medicine, New Haven, Connecticut

ELISABETH M. BATTINELLI, MD, PhD
Assistant Professor of Medicine, Division of Hematology, Brigham and Women's Hospital, Boston, Massachusetts

JORGE J. CASTILLO, MD
Assistant Professor, Division of Hematological Malignancies, Dana-Farber Cancer Institute, Harvard Medical School, Boston, Massachusetts

JOHN CHAPIN, MD
Assistant Professor of Medicine, Department of Medicine, Division of Hematology and Medical Oncology, Weill Cornell Medicine and New York Presbyterian Hospital, New York, New York

NATHAN T. CONNELL, MD, MPH
Division of Hematology, Brigham and Women's Hospital, Harvard Medical School, Boston, Massachusetts

NILANJAN GHOSH, MD, PhD
Chief, Lymphoma Division, Department of Hematologic Oncology and Blood Disorders, Associate Director of Clinical Trials, Levine Cancer Center, Carolinas HealthCare System, Charlotte, North Carolina

STEPHANIE HALENE, MD
Assistant Professor, Section of Hematology, Department of Internal Medicine, Yale Comprehensive Cancer Center, Yale University School of Medicine, New Haven, Connecticut

SHAHRUKH KHURSHID HASHMI, MD, MPH
Assistant Professor of Medicine, Mayo Clinic, Rochester, Minnesota

MARIE A. HOLLENHORST, MD, PhD
Resident, Internal Medicine, Brigham and Women's Hospital, Boston, Massachusetts

ANNA KOVALSZKI, MD
Allergy and Inflammation, Beth Israel Deaconess Medical Center, Instructor of Medicine, Harvard Medical School, Brookline, Massachusetts

ALFRED IAN LEE, MD, PhD
Assistant Professor, Section of Hematology, Yale Cancer Center, Yale University School of Medicine, New Haven, Connecticut

EUN-JU LEE, MD
Assistant Professor, Division of Hematology, Weill Cornell Medical College, New York, New York

EMILIANO N. MUGNAINI, MD, PhD
Physician, Department of Hematologic Oncology and Blood Disorders, Levine Cancer Center, Carolinas HealthCare System, Charlotte, North Carolina

MAUREEN OKAM ACHEBE, MD, MPH
Division of Hematology, Brigham and Women's Hospital; Hematology Services, Dana-Farber Cancer Institute, Assistant Professor, Harvard Medical School, Boston, Massachusetts

CHISOM ONUOHA, MD
St. Mary's Hospital, Waterbury, Connecticut

MARCIA PADDOCK, MD, PhD
Fellow, Department of Medicine, Division of Hematology and Oncology, Weill Cornell Medicine and New York Presbyterian Hospital, New York, New York

ARIC PARNES, MD
Instructor, Division of Hematology, Brigham and Women's Hospital; Dana-Farber Cancer Institute, Boston, Massachusetts

DARRYL J. POWELL, MD
Resident Physician, Department of Medicine, Brigham and Women's Hospital; Department of Pediatrics, Boston Children's Hospital, Boston, Massachusetts

ARVIND RAVI, MD, PhD
Fellow, Dana-Farber Cancer Institute, Boston, Massachusetts

PETER F. WELLER, MD
Beth Israel Deaconess Medical Center, William Bosworth Castle, Professor of Medicine, Harvard Medical School, Boston, Massachusetts

PAGE WIDICK, MD
Department of Internal Medicine, Rhode Island Hospital, Brown University, Providence, Rhode Island

ERIC S. WINER, MD
Associate Professor, Division of Hematology/Oncology, Rhode Island Hospital, Brown University, Providence, Rhode Island

MINA XU, MD
Department of Pathology, Yale University School of Medicine, New Haven, Connecticut

Contents

Anemia denotes a reduced red blood cell (RBC) mass from any cause. The causes of anemia are numerous and due to decreased (or abnormal) erythropoesis, shortened RBC life span, or blood loss. The most common etiology of anemia is iron deficiency. A judicious work up of anemia includes evaluating the reticulocyte count and peripheral smear. The severity of illness of a patient with anemia is determined by the degree of anemia and the seriousness of the underlying disorder. Management of patients with hereditary and hemolytic anemias should involve a hematologist.

Thrombocytopenia is a commonly encountered hematologic problem in inpatient and ambulatory medicine. The many underlying mechanisms of thrombocytopenia include pseudothrombocytopenia, splenic sequestration, and marrow underproduction and destruction. This article presents the known causes of thrombocytopenia, a framework for evaluation, and brief descriptions of management in a case-based format.

Cytopenias are not disease entities in and of themselves; rather, they are the expression of various underlying disease processes. Careful attention to details in patients' presentation, careful history and examination, as well as attention to the ancillary parameters of the complete blood count with a peripheral blood smear can point the clinician toward the appropriate workup. Causes of cytopenias can be inherited or acquired; the latter include medication related, autoimmune, or neoplastic causes. Emergencies need to be recognized in a timely fashion and expert consultation obtained.

Leukocytosis is among the most common findings on peripheral blood smear. A wide range of causes may mediate this finding, and careful clinical and laboratory evaluation assist in differentiating between benign and malignant causes of increased white blood cell counts. In this article, various nonmalignant causes are explored, including infectious, inflamma-tory, autoimmune, and allergic. In addition, malignant causes of leukocy-tosis are discussed, including myeloproliferative disorders, acute leukemia, and chronic leukemia, as well as treatment and monitoring for patients with these diseases.

Myeloproliferative neoplasms (MPNs) are diseases of excess cell prolifer-ation from bone marrow precursors. Two classic MPNs, polycythemia vera (PV) and essential thrombocytosis (ET), are conditions of excess prolifera-tion of red blood cells and platelets, respectively. Although PV and ET involve different cells in the myeloid lineage, their clinical presentations have shared features, consistent with overlapping mutations in growth fac-tor signaling. The management of both diseases involves minimizing the risk of thrombotic and hemorrhagic complications. Both PV and ET can progress to myelofibrosis or acute myeloid leukemia, portending a poor prognosis. MPNs can also present as primary myelofibrosis.

Eosinophilia is defined as elevation of eosinophils in the bloodstream (450–550 cell/μL). There are many reasons for eosinophilia to exist, including parasitic disease, allergic disease, autoimmune, connective tissue disease, rheumatologic disease, primary eosinophilia such as hy-pereosinophilic syndrome, and as part of a malignant state. Primary care physicians should have an understanding of the variety of diseases or sit-uations that can produce eosinophilia and know in what setting referral to specialty care may be warranted.

Patients with derangements of secondary hemostasis resulting from in-herited or acquired thrombophilias are at increased risk of venous throm-boemboli (VTE). Evaluation of a patient with suspected VTE proceeds via evidence-based algorithms that involve computing a pretest probability based on the history and physical examination; this guides subsequent work-up, which can include D dimer and/or imaging. Testing for hyper-coagulable disorders should be pursued only in patients with VTE with an increased risk for an underlying thrombophilia. Direct oral anticoagu-lants are first-line VTE therapies, but they should be avoided in patients who are pregnant, have active cancer, antiphospholipid antibody syn-drome, severe renal insufficiency, or prosthetic heart valves.

Many complex elements contribute to normal hemostasis, and an imbal-ance of these elements may lead to abnormal bleeding. In addition to evaluating medication effects, the hematologist must evaluate for congenital or acquired deficiencies in coagulation factors and platelet disorders. This evaluation should include a thorough bleeding history with careful attention to prior hemostatic challenges and common laboratory testing, including coagulation studies and/or functional platelet assays. An accurate diagnosis of a bleeding diathesis and selection of appropriate treatment are greatly aided by a basic understanding of the mechanisms of disease and the tests used to diagnose them.

Transfusion of various blood components can provide relief from symptomatic anemia and reduce the bleeding risks associated with low platelet counts or presence of coagulopathy. Blood components are collected from volunteer donors and processed into separate components to maximize efficient utilization of a scarce resource while also providing maximum clinical benefit. Tests including blood type and screening for clinically significant alloantibodies increase the likelihood of successful transfusion. Risks of transfusion include hypersensitivity and hemolytic transfusion reactions, transfusion-related acute lung injury, transfusion-associated circulatory overload, and transmission of infection. Indications for transfusion are reviewed along with various products available for transfusion.

Lymphomas may be broadly divided into non-Hodgkin (90%) and Hodgkin (10%) types. Most lymphomas (90%) are of B cell origin but can also be T cell or natural killer cell. Clinical management of indolent and aggressive lymphomas is different. Aggressive lymphomas are more dangerous if left untreated yet a higher cell proliferation rate also renders them more chemosensitive, so they are managed with curative intent. Indolent lymphomas are, for the most part, incurable, such that quality of life must be balanced against toxicity of treatment in deciding when and how to treat.

Plasma cell disorders are benign, premalignant, and malignant conditions characterized by the presence of a monoclonal paraprotein detected in serum or urine. These conditions are biologically, pathologically, and clinically heterogeneous. There have been major advances in the understanding of the biology of these diseases, which are promoting the development of therapies with novel mechanisms of action. Novel agents such as proteasome inhibitors, immunomodulatory drugs, and monoclonal antibodies have gained approval in the United States and Europe for the treatment of plasma cell disorders. Such therapies are translating into higher rates of response and survival and better toxicity profiles.

More than 60,000 hematopoietic cell transplantations (HCTs) are annually
performed worldwide to treat a variety of malignant and nonmalignant conditions. Although HCT is complicated and risky, a majority of the HCT recipients are surviving for many years post-transplant. This article presents
the basics of transplantation, HCT types/stem cell sources, mobilization
and conditioning procedures, indications for HCT, conditioning regimens,
engraftment, graft-versus-host-disease, and survivorship issues.

PRIMARY CARE:
CLINICS IN OFFICE PRACTICE

PRIMARY CARE
CLINICS IN OFFICE PRACTICE

FORTHCOMING ISSUES

March 2017
Primary Care of the Medically Underserved
Vincent Morelli, Roger Zoorob, and
Joel J. Heidelbaugh, Editors

June 2017
Integrative Medicine
Deborah S. Clements and Melinda Ring,
Editors

September 2017
Geriatrics
Demetra Antimisiaris and
Pangkaj Gupta, Editors

RECENT ISSUES

September 2016
Allergy Primer for Primary Care
Michael A. Malone, Editor

June 2016
Psychiatric Care in Primary Care Practice
Janet Albers, Editor

March 2016
Obesity Management in Primary Care
Mark B. Stephens, Editor

ISSUE OF RELATED INTEREST

Hematology/Oncology Clinics of North America
Volume 30, Issue IV, 2016
Imaging of Neurologic Complications in Hematological Disorders
Sangam Kanekar, Editor
Available at: http://www.hemonc.theclinics.com/

THE CLINICS ARE AVAILABLE ONLINE!
Access your subscription at:
www.theclinics.com

Foreword
Strange Cells

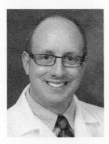

Joel J. Heidelbaugh, MD, FAAFP, FACG
Consulting Editor

With grand aspirations of attending medical school, I was fortunate to land a job in a medical laboratory during my summer vacations when I was in college. Having absolutely no background in medical language and jargon, I felt like I was in a new country and trying to learn a new language. I was fortunate to have a hematopathologist take me under her wing and not only teach me the lingo but also show me hundreds of slides of incredibly strange and fascinating cells. Within a few weeks, I could pronounce and identify the various types of white and red blood cells found in the normal complete blood counts with a differential. However, I was most fascinated with the abnormal and pathologic cases with strange-looking and abnormal numbers of cells. I would soon realize the challenge of interpreting the significance of the results of the slides, without the context of the patient history, physical examination, or medical comorbidities.

This issue of the *Primary Care: Clinics in Office Practice* provides a very detailed overview of many common hematology topics that primary care providers encounter in daily practice as well as those that we commonly worry about missing. The issue commences with a review of anemias and thrombocytopenias, conditions we all routinely see on a weekly basis. Articles with practical guidelines follow, detailing strategies for evaluation and management of conditions with abnormally low or elevated white blood cell counts. Overviews of the various types of leukemia and lymphoma are presented as well as conditions of hypercoagulable states and bleeding diatheses. Guidelines for blood transfusions are presented as well as for bone marrow transplantation. While most primary care providers may not be directing the care of a patient with a neoplastic hematologic disorder, we are likely to be involved in the overall management of these patients as well as in the coordination of care and management of related complications.

I greatly thank Drs Okam and Parnes for their outstanding efforts on this issue of *Primary Care: Clinics in Office Practice*, which was long overdue in its compilation. I would also like to extend my gratitude to our authors and experts who contributed their time and expertise to this issue. As with many of our *Primary Care: Clinics in Office Practice* issues, it is our hope that this will provide a useful reference for you in daily practice.

Joel J. Heidelbaugh, MD, FAAFP, FACG
Departments of Family Medicine and Urology
University of Michigan Medical School
Ann Arbor, MI 48109, USA

Ypsilanti Health Center
200 Arnet Suite 200
Ypsilanti, MI 48198, USA

E-mail address:
jheidel@umich.edu

Preface

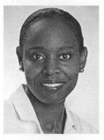 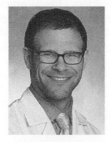

Maureen Okam Achebe,   Aric Parnes, MD
MD, MPH

Editors

The field of Hematology is changing in many exciting ways. Since our time in training, we have seen the advent of new direct oral anticoagulants, targeted therapies in chronic myelogenous leukemia and B-cell lymphomas, and long-acting (and soon even longer duration) factor replacement in hemophilia. We have also seen improved risk stratification, maturing of reduced intensity and haploidentical stem-cell transplant, and the rebirth of gene therapy. These are changes that have improved the quality of life and survival of our patients. Yet, these changes reflect only the tip of the iceberg when we consider the panoply of advances in our knowledge of genetics and pathophysiology, for example, the discovery of a gene (JAK2) responsible for myeloproliferative neoplasms and our clearer understanding of what makes a hematopoetic stem cell metamorphose into the aggressive cell it is in acute myelogenous leukemia.

So, we have brought you a collection of current articles in general hematology that attempts to cover most of what the primary care physician needs to know. Our authors stem from some of the finest academic centers in the country and have addressed key subjects in the field. For example, Dr Okam has written an article about anemia, an important first step for any collection of Hematology. Work on cytopenias continues with reviews on thrombocytopenia and leukopenia/pancytopenia, by Drs Lee and Halene. Then, the opposite problem is tackled with articles on excessive proliferation of cells, including leukocytosis/leukemia, polycythemia, and thrombocytosis, led by Drs Winer and Parnes. Because eosinophilia is so common in general medicine, we felt that eosinophilic disorders deserved its own article. The article in eosinophilia is led by Dr Weller. Rounding out benign hematology, Dr Battinelli brings a pertinent perspective to thrombosis and the recently revamped world of anticoagulation, while Dr Chapin covers the essentials of bleeding disorders. No text on Hematology would be complete without input from Transfusion Medicine, a topic relevant in practically all fields of medicine. Dr Connell addresses important aspects of transfusion in his article. Finally, several topics in malignant hematology are covered, with reviews on lymphoma, multiple myeloma, and stem cell transplantation, by Drs Mugnaini, Castillo, and Hashmi.

Prim Care Clin Office Pract 43 (2016) xv–xvi
http://dx.doi.org/10.1016/j.pop.2016.10.001
0095-4543/16/© 2016 Published by Elsevier Inc.   **primarycare.theclinics.com**

Primary care physicians stand on the frontline of medical care and must be prepared to provide diagnosis, treatment, and appropriate referrals for patients with abnormal blood counts and other hematologic disorders. These articles have been designed to provide some clarity to the critical aspects of hematology. As coeditors, we are grateful for the hard work, expertise, and dedication of our authors. As you go through this journey in Hematology, we hope you will share our enthusiasm.

Maureen Okam Achebe, MD, MPH
Harvard Medical School
Dana Farber Cancer Institute
Hematology Services
Division of Hematology
Brigham and Women's Hospital
Mid-Campus 3
75 Francis Street
Boston, MA 02115, USA

Aric Parnes, MD
Department of Medicine
Division of Hematology
Brigham and Women's Hospital
Dana-Farber Cancer Institute
Harvard Medical School
75 Francis Street
Boston, MA 02115, USA

E-mail addresses:
mokam@bwh.harvard.edu (M.O. Achebe)
aparnes@partners.org (A. Parnes)

Anemia for the Primary Care Physician

Darryl J. Powell, MD[a,b], Maureen Okam Achebe, MD, MPH[c,*]

KEYWORDS

- Anemia • Iron deficiency • Anemia of inflammation • Anemia of chronic disease
- Hemolytic anemia

KEY POINTS

- Anemia is always a sign of an underlying disease or deficiency. Pay attention to identifying the cause. A focused history, physical examination, complete blood cell count, reticulocyte count, and peripheral smear examination are the first steps in a work-up of anemia.
- Iron deficiency is the most common cause of anemia. Repletion of iron stores should be accompanied by identification of the cause of iron deficiency.
- The hallmark of cobalamin deficiency is the presence of neurologic symptoms. Treatment of CNS symptoms should be prompt and parenteral to prevent irreversible damage.
- Anemia of inflammation (AI) is caused by hepcidin-induced alterations of iron metabolism. Besides treating the underlying cause, erythropoietin (EPO)-stimulating agents (ESAs) and intravenous iron are effective in management.
- Hemolytic anemias, whether hereditary or acquired, are frequently chronic problems that require intermittent treatment, at least, and lifelong surveillance. A hematologist is best involved in the management.

INTRODUCTION

The World Health Organization defines anemia as a hemoglobin level of less than 13 g/dL in men and less than 12 g/dL in women. This is based on the average hemoglobin of healthy individuals. **Table 1** shows the World Health Organization limits for anemia defined as mild, moderate, and severe. Unless considered severe, anemia is often overlooked by primary care physicians. It is crucial to appreciate that even mild anemia may be an indication of a serious underlying condition. This article presents anemia and its management as they pertain to the primary care setting.

Disclosure Statement: The authors have nothing to disclose.
[a] Department of Medicine, Brigham and Women's Hospital, Boston, MA, USA; [b] Department of Pediatrics, Children's Hospital, Boston, MA, USA; [c] Division of Hematology, Brigham and Women's Hospital, Harvard Medical School, 75 Francis Street, Midcampus 3, Boston, MA 01701, USA
* Corresponding author.
E-mail address: mokam@bwh.harvard.edu

Prim Care Clin Office Pract 43 (2016) 527–542
http://dx.doi.org/10.1016/j.pop.2016.07.006
0095-4543/16/© 2016 Elsevier Inc. All rights reserved.

primarycare.theclinics.com

Table 1
Anemia severity classification (hemoglobin values in grams per deciliter)

Population	Anemia		
	Mild	Moderate	Severe
Pregnant women	10.0–10.9	7.0–9.9	<7.0
Nonpregnant women (≥15 y of age)	11.0–11.9	8.0–10.9	<8.0
Men (≥15 y of age)	11.0–12.9	8.0–10.9	<8.0

Data from WHO. Haemoglobin concentrations for the diagnosis of anaemia and assessment of severity. Vitamin and mineral nutrition information system. Geneva: World Health Organization; 2011. (WHO/NMH/NHD/MNM/11.1). Available at: http://www.who.int/vmnis/indicators/haemoglobin.pdf. Accessed June 7, 2016.

A broad classification is presented of anemia and details provided for the more common causes of anemia. The rarer diagnoses are touched on briefly and are best referred to a hematologist.

ERYTHROPOIESIS

To understand the etiology of anemia, a basic understanding of erythropoiesis, the process by which red blood cells (RBCs) are produced, is necessary. The primary regulatory hormone involved in erythropoiesis is EPO. This hormone is mostly produced by the kidney (small amounts are produced in the liver) and its release is contingent on the availability of oxygen for tissue metabolic needs. Once released, EPO stimulates both the production and maturation of erythroid precursor cells in the bone marrow. The availability of key nutrients—iron, vitamin B_{12}, and folate—is essential for normal erythropoiesis. Other critical elements of erythropoiesis include a healthy bone marrow and a normal hemoglobin type.

Evaluation of a Patient with Anemia

History
Obtaining a good history is important. Key questions to address in the history include the following:

- Has there been any blood loss?
- What is the duration of the anemia? Is this genetic or acquired?
- Are there associated features? And, therefore, are they due to infection or malignancy?
- Are there comorbidities known to cause anemia (eg, renal failure, rheumatoid arthritis, and inflammatory bowel disease)?
- Does the patient's ethnicity influence the differential?

A thorough medication history, including use of aspirin and nonsteroidal anti-inflammatory drugs, may be useful.[1]

Physical examination
The physical examination helps both confirm the presence of anemia (particularly in low resource settings) and determine the cause. Pallor of the conjunctiva has a sensitivity and specificity of 70% to 100%, respectively. Jaundice in the presence of anemia provides a clue to an etiology of hemolysis.[2]

Other important findings are accompanying lymphadenopathy, hepatosplenomegaly, bone tenderness, petechiae, and ecchymoses.

Laboratory evaluation

The initial laboratory evaluation of anemia is straightforward and involves

- Complete blood cell count with differential
- Reticulocyte count
- Peripheral smear

These 3 tests aid in narrowing the extremely broad differential of anemia and serve as a framework for discussing the various causes of anemia.

The reticulocyte count

The reticulocyte count is a proxy for the ability of the bone marrow to produce new RBCs. The reticulocyte count is a widely available laboratory test that should be used with every evaluation of anemia. It is often reported as a percentage (of RBCs). Although this is useful, a more useful value is the reticulocyte index (RI), which is the reticulocyte count adjusted for the degree of anemia. The RI is calculated as follows:

$$RI = Reticulocyte\ count \cdot \frac{Hematocrit}{Normal\ Hematocrit\ (45)}$$

An RI greater than 2 indicates an appropriate response by the bone marrow to the anemia. The RI distinguishes between a hypoproliferative anemia and an anemia due to blood loss or hemolysis. These are discussed in detail later.

The complete blood cell count and differential returns a whole host of RBC indices. The most important index for the primary care clinician is the mean corpuscular volume (MCV), the average size of the RBCs. The MCV distinguishes between microcytic (MCV <70), normocytic (MCV 70–95), and macrocytic (MCV >95) anemias.

Other laboratory tests useful in the evaluation of anemia are

- Direct and indirect bilirubin
- Lactate dehydrogenase (LDH)
- Haptoglobin

An increase in reticulocyte count, indirect bilirubin, and LDH along with a decrease in haptoglobin are consistent with a hemolytic process.

HYPOPROLIFERATIVE ANEMIA (LOW RETICULOCYTE COUNT)

Anemias with a low reticulocyte, or hypoproliferative anemias, comprise the most common forms of anemia encountered in the primary care setting. These anemias can be further delineated using a morphologic classification based on the size of the RBCs (MCV).

MICROCYTIC ANEMIA
Iron Deficiency Anemia

Iron deficiency is the most common cause of anemia and is estimated to be present in 1% to 2% of the adult population. Iron deficiency in the absence of anemia is present in up to 11% of the adult population.[3] The anemia results from decreased availability of iron for erythropoiesis. In absolute iron deficiency there is a lack of total body iron. In functional iron deficiency, a new term, iron availability, is not sufficient for the intended use, specifically in therapeutic ESA use. This discussion focuses on absolute iron deficiency.

Clinical manifestations

The clinical manifestations of iron deficiency anemia (IDA) are varied. Common symptoms include

- Symptoms of anemia: fatigue, dizziness, headaches, palpitations, and so forth
- Symptoms specific for iron deficiency
  - Pica and/or pagophagia
  - Brittle integument
  - Beeturia
  - Restless leg syndrome (RLS)

Pica is an abnormal appetite for items that are not considered food — sand, clay, starch, raw rice, and so forth. Pagophagia more specifically refers to an insatiable craving for ice. Pagophagia is specific for IDA and is often the first symptom to resolve with the iron supplementation.[4] Beeturia refers to the excretion of red urine after eating beets and occurs in up to 80% of individuals with IDA who eat beets. Beeturia is related to increased intestinal absorption of betanin (red pigmentation of beets), which is normally decolorized by ferric ions.[5]

Signs of iron deficiency are nonspecific and include pallor, cheilosis (fissures at the corners of the mouth), decreased tongue papillation, and koilonychia (spooning of nails).

Restless leg syndrome RLS, or Willis-Ekbom disease, is characterized by a marked discomfort of the lower extremities at rest that is immediately relieved by movement. The pathogenesis of RLS remains poorly understood, although a variety of both central and peripheral nervous system abnormalities are identified in patients. The most consistently implicated central nervous system alteration in patients with RLS is reduced central iron stores: cerebrospinal fluid ferritin is lower than in controls and MRI shows reduced stores in the striatum and red nucleus.[6,7] RLS may be present in up to 24% of individuals with IDA.[8]

Laboratory evaluation

Serum or plasma ferritin Serum or plasma ferritin is the best indicator of the body's iron stores. A ferritin concentration of less than 15 ng/mL is 99% specific for iron deficiency. A low ferritin is easier to interpret than an elevated ferritin because systemic inflammation and hepatocellular injury can lead to increased ferritin levels.

Serum iron Serum iron is typically decreased in iron deficiency but serum iron levels are labile and can be transiently altered by 1 iron-rich meal.

Total iron binding capacity Total iron binding capacity (TIBC), which measures the functional capacity of transferrin to bind iron, is increased in iron deficiency. The (fasting) serum iron and TIBC are used to calculate percent transferrin saturation, which is low (typically <10%) in iron deficiency (**Table 2**). IDA is often accompanied by reactive thrombocytosis.[9]

The peripheral smear The peripheral smear shows hypochromic, microcytic RBCs of varied shape (poikilocytosis) and size (anisocytosis), consistent with a low MCV and an elevated RDW (**Fig. 1**).

Table 2
Laboratory values in iron deficiency and anemia of inflammation

Laboratory Test (Serum/Plasma)	Ferritin	Iron	Total Iron Binding Capacity
Iron deficiency	Decreased	Decreased	Increased
Anemia of inflammation	Normal or increased	Decreased	Decreased

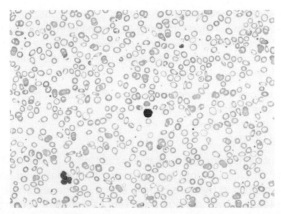

Fig. 1. Iron deficiency. Smear showing microcytic (smaller than the nucleus of a mature lymphocyte), hypochromic (central pallor over one-third of the cell) RBCs. Also showing cells of different shapes (poikilocytosis) (hematoxylin-eosin, original magnification ×50). (*Courtesy of* W.H. Churchill, MD, Brigham and Women's Hospital, Boston, MA.)

The reticulocyte hemoglobin concentration (CHr) is a reflection of recent iron availability for erythropoiesis. CHr is low in iron deficiency as well as in restricted iron availability associated with inflammation. CHr is of limited use and has not been widely adopted in the work-up of iron deficiency. CHr may be useful in patients with end-stage renal disease.[10,11]

Causes of iron-deficiency anemia

Iron deficiency is due to

- Poor dietary intake of iron (mostly in the developing countries)
- Decreased iron absorption
- Increased blood loss (most common cause in the Western world)

IDA should prompt an evaluation for blood loss, usually from the gastrointestinal (GI) tract or the genitourinary tract, particularly in female patients. Patients should undergo testing for GI blood loss via fecal occult blood tests, upper endoscopy, and/or colonoscopy to rule out a GI malignancy. Potential causes of decreased iron absorption should be excluded (**Table 3**).

Table 3 Mechanisms of iron deficiency	
Mechanism of Iron Deficiency	**Examples of Causes**
Decreased iron absorption	Atrophic gastritis Celiac disease Gastric bypass *H pylori* infection Calcium-rich foods Proton pump inhibitors Other medications that decrease gastric acidity
Blood/iron loss	Pulmonary hemosiderosis Intravascular hemolysis Hematuria or hemoglobinuria

Treatment of iron-deficiency anemia

Iron supplementation can be given orally or IV. Frontline iron supplementation is oral replacement, which is often effective, inexpensive, and easy to administer. There are certain cases in which IV iron supplementation may be warranted as first-line therapy and these include

- Ongoing blood loss that exceeds the capacity of the GI tract to absorb iron
- Gastric bypass surgery
- Inflammatory bowel disease
- Intolerance of oral iron

The IV iron formulations currently available in the United States are listed in **Table 4**.

There are many formulations of oral iron currently available for use in the United States and for the most part they are equally effective. The recommended daily dose of iron supplementation for an average adult ranges between 150 mg and 200 mg of elemental iron,[9] although this far surpasses the absorptive capacity of the GI system.

GI side effects are common and often impede adherence. These include constipation (which is dose related), epigastric discomfort (which is not dose dependent and is transient in some patients, lasting only a few days), nausea, and metallic taste. Strategies to decrease side effects include reducing the dose, changing the formulation from tablet to solution, and dietary modification (take with food or milk).

Intravenous iron

With the advent of safer formulations of IV iron than those available in the 1980s, appropriate IV iron use is on the rise. The IV iron formulations currently available in the United States are listed in **Table 4**. Although there is a formula to calculate the exact deficit of iron in an individual, this formula is not routinely used in clinical practice. On average, a patient with IDA requires approximately 1000 mg to 1500 mg of elemental iron for complete supplementation. The side-effect profile of IV irons

Table 4
US Food and Drug Administration–approved intravenous iron formulations

Intravenous Iron Formulation	US Food and Drug Administration Approval Date	Maximum Food and Drug Administration – Approved Dose	Food and Drug Administration– Approved Indications for Use[a]
LMW iron dextran	1991	100 mg[b]	Dialysis-associated anemia
HMW iron dextran	1996	100 mg[b]	Oral iron is impossible for any reason
Ferric gluconate	1999	125 mg	CKD on HD receiving ESA
Iron sucrose	2000	200 mg[b]	All stages of CKD
Ferumoxytol	2009	510 mg	Adults with CKD
Ferric carboxymaltose	2013	750 mg	Adults not tolerating or not responding to oral iron.

Abbreviations: CKD, chronic kidney disease; HD, hemodialysis; HMW, high molecular weight; LMW, low molecular weight.
[a] IV iron formulations are routinely used outside of the strict FDA-approved indications.
[b] Dose used in clinical practice often exceed FDA labeling dose. LMW iron dextran is given at 1000-mg doses and iron sucrose at doses up to 300 mg.

differs completely from that of oral iron. IV irons have few, if any, GI side effects. On the other hand, with IV iron, patients may have infusion reactions, which are not anaphylactic[12] and are easily amenable to acetaminophen and H_2-blocker therapy, although anaphylaxis can rarely occur.

Follow-up
The optimal duration of oral supplementation has not been determined but experts suggest oral supplementation for at least 3 to 6 months before expected normalization of all iron studies.[9]

Anemia of Inflammation

AI (formerly anemia of chronic disease) is the second most common form of anemia, after IDA, previously thought related strictly to an underlying inflammatory, infectious, or malignant process. Many more conditions are now known to cause inflammation and thence AI, such as diabetes mellitus and severe trauma. The major causes of AI include

- Malignancy
- HIV infection
- Rheumatologic disorders
- Inflammatory bowel disease
- Castleman disease
- Heart failure
- Renal insufficiency
- Chronic obstructive pulmonary disease

The etiology of AI is multifactorial and has been linked to hepcidin-induced alterations of iron metabolism leading to decreased iron absorption in the GI tract and iron trapping in macrophages.[13,14] Other abnormalities seen in AI include the following:

- Inability to increase erythropoiesis
- Relative decrease in EPO production
- Decreased red cell survival

The underlying mechanism of these changes is mediated by the release of inflammatory cytokines, tumor necrosis factor α, interleukin (IL)-1, and IL-6, which in turn cause the release of interferon-β and interferon-γ.

Laboratory evaluation
The laboratory tests used to make a diagnosis of AI include a serum iron, TIBC, and ferritin (see **Table 2**). Peripheral smear shows microcytic or normocytic RBCs (normochromic in a majority of cases). Other findings include a normal to increased EPO level, low RI, and normal soluble transferrin receptor level.

Treatment
The primary treatment of AI is treatment of the underlying disorder. IV iron supplementation and EPO administration may be effective; however, referral to a hematologist is recommended.[15]

Other causes of microcytic anemia are listed in **Table 5**.

MACROCYTIC ANEMIA

Macrocytic anemias are divided into megaloblastic and nonmegaloblastic anemias.

Table 5
Other causes of microcytic anemia

Microcytic Anemia	Description
Thalassemia	An inherited disorder of hemoglobin chain synthesis
Sideroblastic anemia	Result from acquired or congenital defects in heme synthesis. Common causes of acquired sideroblastic anemia include lead poisoning, alcohol abuse, copper deficiency, and medications (eg, isoniazid and linezolid).
Myelodysplastic syndrome with acquired thalassemia	A rare phenomenon in which myelodysplastic syndrome leads to abnormal hemoglobin chain synthesis

Megaloblastic Anemia

Megaloblastic anemia results from impaired DNA synthesis, which is commonly caused by folate or cobalamin (vitamin B_{12}) deficiency. Other causes include various chemotherapeutic agents that either impair absorption of vitamin B_{12} and folate or block enzymes involved in DNA synthesis. The peripheral smear shows hypersegmented neutrophils and macro-ovalocytes.

Causes and clinical manifestations

Folate and cobalamin deficiency lead to an identical megaloblastic anemia; however, other clinical manifestations are quite different. The hallmark of cobalamin deficiency is the presence of neurologic symptoms, including, but not limited, to the following:

- Subacute combined degeneration of the dorsal and lateral columns (specific)
- Cerebellar ataxia
- Axonal degeneration of peripheral nerves
- Memory loss
- Dementia

Folate deficiency is related to poor nutrition and decreased intake of folate-rich foods. This is uncommon in the Western world because many foods are fortified with folate.

Vitamin B_{12} is found exclusively in animal protein. Vitamin B_{12} deficiency may be caused by pernicious anemia; autoantibodies against intrinsic factor, which is required for the proper absorption of cobalamin[16]; or other gastric disease or disruption (such as in gastric bypass surgery). Vitamin B_{12} deficiency is less likely due to inadequate dietary intake with the exception of strict vegans. Other causes include chronic proton pump inhibitor or H_2-blocker use, HIV, and *Helicobacter pylori* infection.[17–19]

Laboratory evaluation

The first step involves the measurement of serum folate and cobalamin concentrations. If these tests are equivocal (low normal) and deficiency is suspected, the next step is metabolite testing, measuring methylmalonic acid and homocysteine. Methylmalonic acid and homocysteine are elevated in vitamin B_{12} deficiency, whereas only homocysteine is elevated in folate deficiency. If pernicious anemia is suspected, measurement of intrinsic factor antibodies should be obtained. The classic 2-stage Schilling test using radiolabeled vitamin B_{12} to measure absorption is no longer necessary.[20]

Treatment of folate and cobalamin deficiency

Folate deficiency is treated with 1 mg/d of folate for 1 to 4 months or until hematologic recovery is achieved.

Pernicious anemia is typically treated with parenteral (intramuscularly or subcutaneously) vitamin B_{12}, given 1000 µg daily for 1 week followed by 1000 µg weekly for

4 weeks followed by 1000 μg monthly for life. Oral vitamin B_{12} treatment is often sufficient to treat deficiency in pernicious anemia. Vitamin B_{12}, 1000 μg orally given daily, is absorbed by mass action, not relying on the action of intrinsic factor. Cobalamin deficiency due to other causes is treated with oral vitamin B_{12}, 1000 μg or 2000 μg daily.[21]

Macrocytic Nonmegaloblastic Anemia

Common causes of macrocytosis (not associated with megaloblastosis) include

- Alcohol abuse (in the absence of vitamin B_{12} or folate deficiency)
- Myelodysplastic syndrome
- Liver disease
- Hypothyroidism
- Drugs (hydroxyurea, antiretrovirals, azathioprine, etc.)
- Reticulocytosis

NORMOCYTIC ANEMIAS

Normocytic anemias include a broad array of anemias of normal MCV that may be either hypoproliferative or hyperproliferative. There is considerable overlap between etiologies that cause normocytic, microcytic, and macrocytic anemias (**Table 6**).

Table 6 Common normocytic anemias	
Normocytic Anemias (Normal Mean Corpuscular Volume)	**Overlap with Microcytosis/Macrocytosis**
Acute blood loss	Chronic blood loss causes microcytic anemia
Renal failure	
Hypothyroidism	Severe hypothyroidism may present with macrocytic anemia
Iron deficiency (in early stages of anemia)	Iron deficiency in later stages is microcytic
Anemia of Inflammation	May also be microcytic
Sickle cell anemia	Double heterozygous inheritance of sickle gene with another abnormal gene (eg, thalassemia gene or hemoglobin C) results in microcytosis.

HYPERPROLIFERATIVE/REGENERATIVE ANEMIAS

Hyperproliferative anemias, outside of blood loss, should generally prompt referral to a hematologist because the management of these anemias is often complicated and likely outside the scope of general internal medicine. Hyperproliferative anemias are the result of acute blood loss or increased RBC destruction (hemolysis), which may be due to congenital or acquired causes.

Congenital Hemolytic Anemias

Congenital hemolytic anemias are due to defects in 1 of the following:

- RBC membrane
- RBC metabolism
- RBC hemoglobin

A brief discussion of the most common conditions follows.

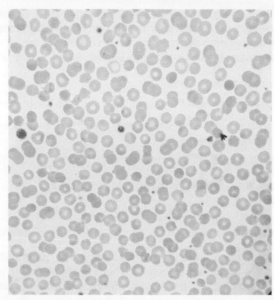

Fig. 2. HS. Smear showing numerous spherocytes (cells with no central pallor) (hematoxylin-eosin, original magnification ×50). (*Courtesy of* W.H. Churchill, MD, Brigham and Women's Hospital, Boston, MA.)

Defects in red cell membrane

Hereditary spherocytosis Hereditary spherocytosis (HS) is the most common hemolytic anemia due to a defect in the RBC membrane, with an incidence of approximately 200 to 300 per million. HS is due to a mutation in genes responsible for the structural proteins (mostly ankyrin and spectrin) of the RBC membrane. These mutations lead to increased fragility of the RBCs, which are more easily destroyed when traversing the spleen. Anemia, jaundice, splenomegaly, and bilirubin stones are characteristic. Because of the shortened lifespan of the RBC, patients are at risk for red cell aplasia when exposed to parvovirus B19.[22]

Laboratory evaluation The most helpful RBC index in making a diagnosis of HS is the mean corpuscular hemoglobin concentration. A majority of patients with HS have a mean corpuscular hemoglobin concentration of greater than or equal to 39 g/dL. The peripheral smear shows spherocytes (**Fig. 2**).

The classic test for HS is the osmotic fragility test, which literally tests for release of hemoglobin from red cells at increasingly dilute salt concentrations. This is no longer widely used because the eosin-5-maleimide binding test, a flow cytometric test, which shows decreased staining of a major RBC membrane structural protein, band 3 protein, in HS, is now the gold standard. It carries an approximately 95% specificity and sensitivity.[23]

Treatment Many cases of HS can be treated with supportive care, including folic acid supplementation and occasional RBC transfusions. For severe cases, splenectomy decreases hemolysis.

Defects in red blood cell metabolism

Glucose-6-phosphate dehydrogenase deficiency Glucose-6-phosphate dehydrogenase (G6PD) deficiency, the most common RBC enzyme disorder, is an X-linked disorder, affecting approximately 400 million people worldwide. G6PD is involved in the pentose phosphate shunt, which allows cells to deal with oxidative stress. RBCs deficient in G6PD are prone to sudden destruction after exposure to drugs with a high redox potential, selected infections, fava beans, and metabolic abnormalities.

The most clinically relevant complication of G6PD deficiency is severe hemolysis after exposure to certain medications. The G6PD Deficiency Favism Association Web site has an extensive list of medications that are considered unsafe in this population: http://www.g6pd.org/en/G6PDDeficiency/SafeUnsafe/DaEvitare_ISS-it.

G6PD deficiency should be considered in a patient presenting with a nonimmune hemolytic anemia after exposure to stress or certain medications. Bite cells or Heinz bodies may be seen on a peripheral smear. The diagnosis is confirmed by measurement of G6PD activity, which should be assessed at least 3 months after a hemolytic episode. The mainstay of treatment is the avoidance of precipitating agents.

Defects in red blood cell hemoglobin (hemoglobinopathies)

Sickle cell disease Sickle cell disease (SCD) is a term encompassing a group of inherited disorders that result from a single base pair mutation in which valine is substituted for glutamic acid as the 6th amino acid in the beta globin chain. This substitution causes sickle hemoglobin to polymerize and RBCs to sickle, or form a crescent shape, when exposed to hypoxic or acidotic conditions. These sickle cells are less flexible and easily occlude small vessels leading to vaso-occlusive crises, characterized by significant pain. Major complications of SCD include cerebrovascular events, asplenia, cardiomegaly and anemic heart failure, pulmonary hypertension and acute chest syndrome, renal failure, and priapism. Greater than 90% of patients with SCD survive into adulthood and require high-quality adult primary care.[24]

Diagnosis of Sickle Cell Disease Universal newborn screening for SCD in the United States has been in effect only since 2008. Therefore, it cannot be assumed that every adult has been screened or diagnosed of this disease. This is particularly true in the developing world where screening is not widely available.[25] The diagnosis of SCD is achieved by one of several methods — isoelectric focusing, hemoglobin electrophoresis, and high-performance liquid chromatography — which identifies the abnormal hemoglobin that differs from normal hemoglobin by charge. Additionally, these methods are able to differentiate homozygous SCD (HbSS, sickle cell anemia) from double heterozygous inheritance of the sickle gene and other abnormal hemoglobins (eg, HbSC, HbSD, Hb S/β-thalassemia, and HbSO-Arab). The peripheral smear shows sickle cells (**Fig. 3**).

Clinical manifestations SCD affects many organ systems and has clinical manifestations that are both acute and chronic in nature.

Most common acute complications of SCD include

- Vaso-occlusive phenomena
  - Acute pain crisis — the hallmark of SCD
  - Acute chest syndrome
  - Stroke
  - Bone infarction/dactylitis
  - Renal infarction
  - Priapism
- Severe anemia
  - Primarily from chronic hemolysis; also during aplastic crisis (parvovirus B19) and hypersplenism before autosplenectomy by adulthood
- Infections
  - Functional asplenia causes vulnerability to encapsulated organisms.

Chronic manifestations of SCD include

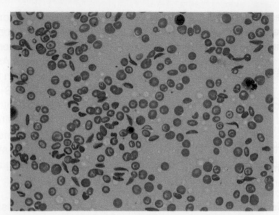

Fig. 3. SCD. Smear showing sickle (shaped) cells, target cells, reticulocytes (the larger cells with a *purple tinge*), and a nucleated RBC in the center of the field (hematoxylin-eosin, original magnification ×50). (*Courtesy of* W.H. Churchill, MD, Brigham and Women's Hospital, Boston, MA.)

- Chronic anemia
- Pulmonary hypertension
- Chronic kidney disease
- Silent brain infarcts with neurologic deficits
- Cardiomyopathy from chronic anemia
- Iron overload (from chronic transfusions)
- Chronic leg ulcers
- Proliferative retinopathy

Treatment of sickle cell disease The mainstay of chronic treatment of SCD is hydroxyurea, which increases fetal hemoglobin. Hydroxyurea causes bone marrow suppression and forces stress erythropoiesis that is accompanied by induction of fetal hemoglobin. Fetal hemoglobin disrupts polymer formation of sickle hemoglobin. Hydroxyurea decreases the frequency of painful episodes, acute chest syndrome, and severe symptomatic anemia. Hydroxyurea causes macrocytosis and neutropenia. These can be used as markers of adherence.

RBC exchange transfusions are administered to decrease the percent sickle hemoglobin in the blood while maintaining a hematocrit not greater than 33%. The absolute indications for a red cell exchange transfusion include (1) acute chest syndrome[26] and (2) stroke or stroke in evolution (waxing and waning neurologic symptoms). Relative indications for an RBC exchange transfusion include (1) multiorgan failure and (2) sickle cell hepatopathy.

Hematopoietic stem cell transplantation is the only known cure for the disease. As safer conditioning regimens are developed, and the risk-benefit ratio continues to improve, this has the potential to become suitable for more patients with SCD.[27]

Important note: sickle cell trait is a benign carrier condition; however, some studies have suggested an increased risk of sudden death during extreme exercise.[28]

Thalassemia syndromes

The thalassemia syndromes are a heterogeneous group of disorders that result from a defect in production of either the alpha or beta globin chain of hemoglobin. Anemia develops from chronic hemolysis and ineffective erythropoiesis. These syndromes include

β-Thalassemia Results from more than 400 mutations of the beta globin chain. The clinical syndromes are based on signs and symptoms. A hematologist should be involved in the care of all patients with β-thalassemia major or β-thalassemia intermedia.

β-Thalassemia major This is defined by the obligate need for transfusions to maintain livelihood. Patients are transfused RBCs on a routine basis to provide oxygen-carrying capacity and suppress endogenous erythropoiesis.

Diagnosed in childhood and treatment involves chronic transfusion therapy. In the absence of routine chelation therapy, this leads to iron overload and subsequent endocrine, cardiac, and hepatic complications.

β-Thalassemia minor (trait) Often asymptomatic and diagnosed after the incidental finding of hypochromic, microcytic RBCs. No treatment is required.

β-Thalassemia intermedia The range of symptoms varies widely. Patients are variably anemic and icteric. Patients may intermittently need RBC transfusions at times of stress (eg, pregnancy).

These patients do not require transfusion in the first few years of life, but the transfusion need may increase with advancing age. As a result of ineffective erythropoiesis, patients often develop iron overload.

α-Thalassemia Results from mutations of the alpha chain. The clinical syndromes are based on the number of alpha globin deletions.

α-Thalassemia minima The result of missing 1 of 4 alpha globin genes ($-\alpha/\alpha\ \alpha$)
Completely asymptomatic but important for genetic counseling

α-Thalassemia minor The result of missing 2 of 4 alpha globin genes ($-\alpha/-\alpha$) or ($--/\alpha\ \alpha$)
Individuals may have a mild microcytic anemia similar to β-thalassemia trait.

Hemoglobin H (α-thalassemia intermedia) Beta globin tetramers, the result of missing 3 of 4 alpha globin genes ($--/-\alpha$)
Present during gestation and manifests with neonatal jaundice and chronic hemolytic anemia for which patients may not need transfusions until the second or third decade of life.
Can be acquired in certain myelodysplastic syndromes

Hemoglobin Barts (hydrops fetalis) Missing 4 of 4 alpha globin genes ($--/--$)
Universally fatal within hours of birth

Hemoglobin constant spring Common in certain Asian populations

Important note: although β-thalassemia can be diagnosed with hemoglobin electrophoresis, α-thalassemia requires DNA analysis to make the diagnosis.[29]

ACQUIRED HEMOLYTIC ANEMIA

Acquired hemolytic anemias can be classified as immune or nonimmune.

Immune Mediated

Warm autoimmune hemolytic anemia
Warm autoimmune hemolytic anemia (AIHA) is most often due to the development of IgG antibodies that react with protein antigens on the RBC surface, leading to the

destruction of these RBCs as they pass through the spleen. Although most of these causes are idiopathic, some underlying causes include[30]

- Viral infections
- Autoimmune and connective tissue disease
- Immune deficiency
- Malignancy (particularly in chronic lymphocytic leukemia)

Laboratory evaluation
Anemia in the presence of elevated LDH, indirect bilirubin, and decreased haptoglobin should raise suspicion for hemolytic anemia.

AIHA is confirmed by the presence of a positive direct Coombs test, which is present in greater than 95% of patients with warm AIHA.[31]

The peripheral smear shows spherocytes.

Treatment
The mainstay of treatment of AIHA is immunosuppression with either glucocorticoids or biologic agents, such as rituximab (monoclonal antibody against CD20 [B cells]). Splenectomy is done in patients with refractory disease.[32]

Non–immune Mediated

Microangiopathic hemolytic anemia
The presence of hemolytic anemia should always prompt evaluation for a microangiopathic hemolytic anemia (MAHA) or thrombotic microangiopathy. Schistocytes on a peripheral smear are highly suggestive of MAHA. MAHA includes several disorders that require emergent hematology intervention.

- Thombotic thrombocytopenic purpura
  - Pentad of fever, anemia, thrombocytopenia, renal dysfunction, and neurologic symptoms
- Atypical hemolytic uremic syndrome
  - Clinical manifestations: anemia, thrombocytopenia, profound renal dysfunction
- Disseminated intravascular coagulation
  - Clinical manifestations: anemia, thrombocytopenia, decreased fibrinogen, elevated prothrombin time/partial thromboplastin time

Drug-induced hemolytic anemia
Drug-induced hemolytic anemia is rare. Millions of doses of drugs are given to patients without hemolytic anemia occurring. Drug-dependent antibodies, when present, however, may react by multiple methods causing hemolysis. Medications can cause RBC destruction through both immune and nonimmune mechanisms.[33] **Table 7** provides a summary of mechanisms of drug-induced hemolytic anemia.

Table 7
Drug-induced hemolytic anemia

	Mechanism	Prototype Drugs
Nonimmune	Drug-induced oxidative stress (not limited to patients with G6PD deficiency)	Dapsone, nitrites, rifampin
Immune	Immune complex (innocent bystander)	Quinidine, phenacetin
	Drug adsorption (Hapten)	Penicillin
	Nonimmunologic protein adsorption	Cephalothin
	AIHA	Methyldopa

REFERENCES

1. Hung OL, Kwon NS, Cole AE, et al. Evaluation of the physician's ability to recognize the presence or absence of anemia, fever, and jaundice. Acad Emerg Med 2000;7(2):146–56.
2. Sheth TN, Choudhry NK, Bowes M, et al. The relation of conjunctival pallor to the presence of anemia. J Gen Intern Med 1997;12(2):102–6.
3. Looker AC, Dallman PR, Carroll MD, et al. Prevalence of iron deficiency in the United States. JAMA 1997;277(12):973–6.
4. Reynolds RD, Binder HJ, Miller MB, et al. Pagophagia and iron deficiency anemia. Ann Intern Med 1968;69(3):435–40.
5. Sotos JG. Beeturia and iron absorption. Lancet 1999;354(9183):1032.
6. Earley CJ, Connor JR, Beard JL, et al. Abnormalities in CSF concentrations of ferritin and transferrin in restless legs syndrome. Neurology 2000;54(8):1698–700.
7. Rizzo G, Manners D, Testa C, et al. Low brain iron content in idiopathic restless legs syndrome patients detected by phase imaging. Mov Disord 2013;28(13):1886–90.
8. Allen RP, Auerbach S, Bahrain H, et al. The prevalence and impact of restless legs syndrome on patients with iron deficiency anemia. Am J Hematol 2013;88(4):261–4.
9. Auerbach M, Adamson JW. How we diagnose and treat iron deficiency anemia. Am J Hematol 2016;91(1):31–8.
10. Brugnara C, Zurakowski D, DiCanzio J, et al. Reticulocyte hemoglobin content to diagnose iron deficiency in children. JAMA 1999;281(23):2225–30.
11. Fishbane S, Galgano C, Langley RC, et al. Reticulocyte hemoglobin content in the evaluation of iron status of hemodialysis patients. Kidney Int 1997;52(1):217–22.
12. Okam MM, Mandell E, Hevelone N, et al. Comparative rates of adverse events with different formulations of intravenous iron. Am J Hematol 2012;87(11):E123–4.
13. Weiss G, Goodnough LT. Anemia of chronic disease. N Engl J Med 2005;352(10):1011–23.
14. Gangat N, Wolanskyj AP. Anemia of chronic disease. Semin Hematol 2013;50(3):232–8.
15. Cullis JO. Diagnosis and management of anaemia of chronic disease: current status. Br J Haematol 2011;154(3):289–300.
16. Balcı YI, Ergin A, Karabulut A, et al. Serum vitamin B12 and folate concentrations and the effect of the Mediterranean diet on vulnerable populations. Pediatr Hematol Oncol 2014;31(1):62–7.
17. Marcuard SP, Albernaz L, Khazanie PG. Omeprazole therapy causes malabsorption of cyanocobalamin (vitamin B12). Ann Intern Med 1994;120(3):211–5.
18. Remacha AF, Cadafalch J. Cobalamin deficiency in patients infected with the human immunodeficiency virus. Semin Hematol 1999;36(1):75–87.
19. Sumner AE, Chin MM, Abrahm JL, et al. Elevated methylmalonic acid and total homocysteine levels show high prevalence of vitamin B12 deficiency after gastric surgery. Ann Intern Med 1996;124(5):469–76.
20. Green R, Kinsella LJ. Current concepts in the diagnosis of cobalamin deficiency. Neurology 1995;45(8):1435–40.
21. Eussen SJ, de Groot LC, Clarke R, et al. Oral cyanocobalamin supplementation in older people with vitamin B12 deficiency: a dose-finding trial. Arch Intern Med 2005;165(10):1167–72.

22. Cynober T, Mohandas N, Tchernia G. Red cell abnormalities in hereditary spherocytosis: relevance to diagnosis and understanding of the variable expression of clinical severity. J Lab Clin Med 1996;128(3):259–69.
23. Kar R, Mishra P, Pati HP. Evaluation of eosin-5-maleimide flow cytometric test in diagnosis of hereditary spherocytosis. Int J Lab Hematol 2010;32(1 Pt 2):8–16.
24. Bunn HF. Pathogenesis and treatment of sickle cell disease. N Engl J Med 1997; 337(11):762–9.
25. Odame I. Developing a global agenda for sickle cell disease: report of an international symposium and workshop in Cotonou, Republic of Benin. Am J Prev Med 2010;38(4 Suppl):S571–5.
26. Vichinsky EP, Neumayr LD, Earles AN, et al. Causes and outcomes of the acute chest syndrome in sickle cell disease. National acute chest syndrome study group. N Engl J Med 2000;342(25):1855–65.
27. Hsieh MM, Fitzhugh CD, Tisdale JF. Allogeneic hematopoietic stem cell transplantation for sickle cell disease: the time is now. Blood 2011;118(5):1197–207.
28. Kark JA, Posey DM, Schumacher HR, et al. Sickle-cell trait as a risk factor for sudden death in physical training. N Engl J Med 1987;317(13):781–7.
29. Martin A, Thompson AA. Thalassemias. Pediatr Clin North Am 2013;60(6): 1383–91.
30. Gehrs BC, Friedberg RC. Autoimmune hemolytic anemia. Am J Hematol 2002; 69(4):258–71.
31. Sachs UJH, Röder L, Santoso S, et al. Does a negative direct antiglobulin test exclude warm autoimmune haemolytic anaemia? A prospective study of 504 cases. Br J Haematol 2006;132(5):655–6.
32. Petz LD. Treatment of autoimmune hemolytic anemias. Curr Opin Hematol 2001; 8(6):411–6.
33. Mayer B, Bartolmäs T, Yürek S, et al. Variability of findings in drug-induced immune haemolytic anaemia: experience over 20 years in a single centre. Transfus Med Hemother 2015;42(5):333–9.

Thrombocytopenia

Eun-Ju Lee, MD[a], Alfred Ian Lee, MD, PhD[b],*

KEYWORDS

- Thrombocytopenia • Immune thrombocytopenia
- Heparin-induced thrombocytopenia • Thrombotic thrombocytopenia purpura
- Atypical hemolytic uremic syndrome

KEY POINTS

- Major causes of isolated thrombocytopenia include immune thrombocytopenia, drug-induced thrombocytopenia, disseminated intravascular coagulation, heparin-induced thrombocytopenia, gestational thrombocytopenia, and inherited thrombocytopenias.
- Patients with mild, chronic, isolated thrombocytopenia often maintain a platelet count in the range of 100 to 150 × 10⁹/L, whereas some develop immune thrombocytopenia with or without a concomitant autoimmune disease.
- Immune thrombocytopenia is a diagnosis of exclusion and requires evaluation for secondary causes of thrombocytopenia.
- Diagnosis and management of heparin-induced thrombocytopenia rely on an assessment of pretest probability of having this disease.
- Microangiopathic hemolytic anemia and schistocytes are defining features of thrombotic microangiopathies.

INTRODUCTION

Platelets are derived from megakaryocytes whose production and maturation in the bone marrow are regulated by thrombopoietin.[1] Platelets play important roles not only in thrombosis and wound repair but also in inflammation, immunity, and cancer biology.[2] Normal platelet values range from 150 to 450 × 10⁹/L. There is some debate as to whether patients with platelet counts in the range 100 × 10⁹/L to 150 × 10⁹/L should be designated as having true versus borderline thrombocytopenia[3]; data suggest that most of these patients remain asymptomatic and maintain their platelet counts in this range, whereas a smaller percentage develop immune thrombocytopenia (ITP) with or without a concomitant autoimmune disease.[4]

Disclosure: The authors have nothing to disclose.
[a] Division of Hematology, Weill Cornell Medical College, New York, NY, USA; [b] Section of Hematology, Yale Cancer Center, Yale University School of Medicine, 333 Cedar Street, Box 208021, New Haven, CT 06520, USA
* Corresponding author.
E-mail address: alfred.lee@yale.edu

Prim Care Clin Office Pract 43 (2016) 543–557
http://dx.doi.org/10.1016/j.pop.2016.07.008
0095-4543/16/© 2016 Elsevier Inc. All rights reserved.

primarycare.theclinics.com

A major clinical consequence of thrombocytopenia is bleeding caused by impaired primary hemostasis and platelet plug formation. Mucocutaneous bleeding usually occurs when platelet counts decrease to less than the range of 20×10^9/L to 30×10^9/L. Severe bleeding, including intracranial hemorrhage, occurs with platelet counts of less than 10×10^9/L to 20×10^9/L.[5–7]

Thrombocytopenia is a common problem, affecting 40% to 50% of patients in medical and surgical intensive care units.[8–10] In the outpatient setting, primary care physicians are generally comfortable managing patients with at least modest thrombocytopenia (eg, platelet count 80×10^9/L) without referral to a hematologist, so an understanding of the major mechanisms of thrombocytopenia is essential for practicing internists.[11] However, the evaluation of thrombocytopenia can be challenging, because hematologists confronted with the same case of thrombocytopenia frequently disagree on the underlying diagnosis.[12]

The major underlying mechanisms of thrombocytopenia include pseudothrombocytopenia, splenic sequestration, marrow underproduction, and peripheral destruction (**Box 1**). Clues from a patient's history (including medication exposures, alcohol intake, diet, travel, recent illnesses, and transfusions), physical examination (eg, petechiae, mucosal bleeding, splenomegaly, lymphadenopathy, and skeletal abnormalities), family history, and other laboratory studies may refine the differential diagnosis. Of central importance is the peripheral blood smear to evaluate both for the presence of platelet clumps, indicating pseudothrombocytopenia (**Fig. 1**), and for other abnormal cell morphologies, such as schistocytes, large or giant platelets, or immature or dysplastic cells.

This article presents 4 clinical cases as examples of our diagnostic approach to patients with thrombocytopenia.

Case 1

A 20-year-old male college student presented to his university urgent care clinic 3 weeks ago with fever, chills, sore throat, and headache. He was diagnosed with an upper respiratory tract infection. He now returns with epistaxis and gum bleeding. He does not take any medications, vitamins, or herbal supplements. He denies alcohol or recreational drug use. He consumes a broad diet. There is no known family history of cytopenias or other blood disorders. Physical examination reveals wet purpura in the oral cavity, mild crusted blood in the nares, and petechiae on both legs, with no lymphadenopathy or hepatosplenomegaly. Laboratory studies show a white blood cell (WBC) count of 4,400/μL, hemoglobin level 14.4 g/dL, platelet count 1×10^9/L, and preserved coagulation studies (prothrombin time [PT], International Normalized Ratio [INR], and partial thromboplastin time [PTT]). The peripheral blood smear is shown in **Fig. 2**. What is the patient's diagnosis, and how should he be treated?

Petechiae and mucocutaneous bleeding can be seen with platelet disorders, mild coagulation factor deficiencies, or connective tissue disorders. This patient's severe thrombocytopenia and normal coagulation parameters suggest a platelet disorder. Given that the WBC count and hemoglobin are preserved, the evaluation should focus on causes of isolated thrombocytopenia, namely ITP, drug-induced ITP (DITP), disseminated intravascular coagulation (DIC), heparin-induced thrombocytopenia (HIT), gestational thrombocytopenia, and inherited thrombocytopenias.[13] The finding of large or giant platelets on the blood smear suggests either a component of peripheral destruction leading to megakaryocyte hyperplasia in the bone marrow or a platelet structural defect as may be seen in inherited thrombocytopenias; the negative family history points away from the latter. Lack of medication or drug exposure or herbal use renders DITP and HIT unlikely. The absence of systemic symptoms or schistocytes

Box 1
Major mechanisms of thrombocytopenia

Pseudothrombocytopenia

- EDTA (ethylenediamine tetraacetic acid) dependent

Sequestration

- Splenomegaly (portal hypertension)

Bone marrow underproduction

- Infections (Epstein-Barr virus, cytomegalovirus, hepatitis C, human immunodeficiency virus, parvovirus B19, *H pylori*)

- Medications/drugs (antibiotics, alcohol, chemotherapy, radiation)

- Nutritional deficiencies (folate, vitamin B_{12})

- Liver disease

- Bone marrow failure syndromes (aplastic anemia, Fanconi anemia, dyskeratosis congenita, Diamond-Blackfan anemia, Shwachman-Diamond syndrome)

- Hematologic disorders (lymphoma, leukemia, myelodysplastic syndrome)

- Tumor infiltration of bone marrow

- Inherited thrombocytopenias (Bernard-Soulier syndrome, gray platelet syndrome, congenital amegakaryocytic thrombocytopenia, Wiskott-Aldrich syndrome, thrombocytopenia with absent radii, MYH9-related thrombocytopenia)

Increased platelet destruction

- ITP

- Drug-induced ITP (quinine, NSAIDs, glycoprotein IIb/IIIa inhibitors)

- Heparin-induced thrombocytopenia

- TTP/HUS

- Atypical HUS

- Medication-induced TTP (mitomycin C, gemcitabine, oxaliplatin)

- Disseminated intravascular coagulation

- Posttransfusion purpura

- [a]Autoimmune-related thrombocytopenia (SLE, CVID, antiphospholipid antibody syndrome, thyroid disease, Evans syndrome)

- Mechanical destruction (cardiopulmonary bypass, intra-aortic balloon pump)

Abbreviations: CVID, common variable immunodeficiency; HUS, hemolytic uremic syndrome; MYH, myosin heavy chain; NSAIDs, nonsteroidal antiinflammatory drugs; SLE, systemic lupus erythematosus; TTP, thrombotic thrombocytopenic purpura.
[a] Secondary ITP, multiple mechanisms of thrombocytopenia.

and the normal coagulation studies exclude DIC. The most plausible explanation for this patient's severe, isolated thrombocytopenia is therefore ITP.

ITP is an autoimmune disorder caused by antibodies directed against antigens on the surfaces of platelets and megakaryocytes, leading to platelet destruction.[14] Genetic susceptibility in combination with environmental factors (including viral and bacterial infections) may trigger flares of ITP.[15] Despite exhaustive efforts, no disease-causing autoantibody with reliable diagnostic utility has been identified.[16,17]

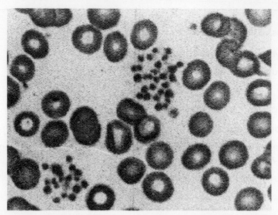

Fig. 1. Pseudothrombocytopenia; this is an in-vitro phenomenon arising from antibodies directed against platelet surface epitopes in the presence of the calcium-chelating agent EDTA (ethylenediamine tetraacetic acid). Measurement of platelet counts using heparin or citrate as the anticoagulant corrects this problem, which is generally of no clinical consequence (hematoxylin-eosin, original magnification ×100). (*From* Shalev O, Lotman A. Images in clinical medicine. Pseudothrombocytopenia. N Engl J Med 1993;329(20):1467; with permission.)

Bone marrow findings in patients with ITP are heterogeneous, rendering the diagnostic utility of this test limited.[18] A diagnosis of ITP therefore remains one of exclusion (see **Box 1**).

ITP may be primary (ie, isolated or idiopathic) or secondary, occurring in the context of other conditions associated with immune dysregulation, such as chronic infections or autoimmune disorders (**Table 1**).[19,20] Clinical manifestations range from mild bruising to severe mucosal bleeding. The risk of bleeding usually correlates with the

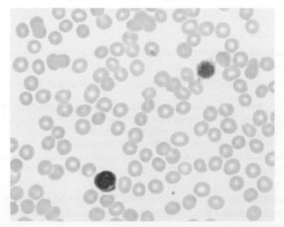

Fig. 2. Peripheral blood smear for case 1. The large cell represents a giant platelet, defined as a platelet of a size similar to a red blood cell. Typically, the smear in ITP shows thrombocytopenia with enlarged or giant platelets, although a smear with strictly giant platelets in the context of a family history of thrombocytopenia should alternatively raise suspicion for an inherited thrombocytopenic disorder (hematoxylin-eosin, original magnification ×100).

Table 1
Causes and evaluation of secondary ITP

Associated Conditions	Recommended Testing
Common variable immunodeficiency	Quantitative immunoglobulins
Evans syndrome	Direct antiglobulin test
Infections	H pylori, human immunodeficiency virus, hepatitis C, [a]parvovirus, [a]cytomegalovirus serologies
Antiphospholipid antibody syndrome	[a]Lupus anticoagulant, anticardiolipin antibodies, anti–beta-2 glycoprotein-1 antibodies
Thyroid disease	[a]Thyroid function tests, antithyroid antibodies
[b]Pregnancy	[a]Pregnancy testing
Systemic lupus erythematosus	[a]ANA

Abbreviation: ANA, antinuclear antibody.
[a] Tests of potential benefit per international consensus guidelines.
[b] In women of childbearing age.
Adapted from Provan D, Stasi R, Newland AC, et al. International consensus report on the investigation and management of primary immune thrombocytopenia. Blood 2010;115(2):169.

degree of thrombocytopenia,[21] although increasingly a risk of thrombosis in patients with severe ITP has been recognized.[22]

Once a diagnosis of ITP is considered, clinicians should perform additional testing to exclude causes of secondary ITP. These causes include quantitative immunoglobulins to evaluate for common variable immunodeficiency (CVID), direct antiglobulin test (direct Coombs test) for Evans syndrome (the combination of ITP and autoimmune hemolytic anemia), and serologies for Helicobacter pylori, human immunodeficiency virus, and hepatitis C.[23] Identifying such conditions may affect treatment, because antimicrobial therapy may lead to hematologic recovery in cases of ITP caused by chronic infections, whereas lower doses or shorter courses of steroids and other immune suppression may be indicated in patients with ITP with CVID to mitigate infectious risk.[20,24–27]

Treatment is recommended for patients with newly diagnosed ITP whose platelet counts are less than 20×10^9/L to 30×10^9/L, or who are bleeding or have upcoming surgical procedures.[28] First-line treatment is corticosteroids, most commonly prednisone (1 mg/kg daily until platelet recovery, followed by a taper) or dexamethasone (40 mg daily for 4 days), with a recent clinical trial suggesting faster hematologic recovery with the latter.[29] Methylprednisolone (30 mg/kg daily for 7 days) is sometimes administered in more severe cases. Initial response rates for all of these interventions are around 70% to 80%, with a time to response ranging from about 2 days to 2 weeks, and variable response duration.[23,28] In patients with severe thrombocytopenia and bleeding, intravenous immunoglobulin (1 g/kg/d for 1–2 days) or, in Rh(D)+ patients, anti-D immunoglobulin (50–70 μg/kg for 1 dose) may be supplemented with steroids, leading to more rapid count recovery.[23,30] Platelet transfusions are generally not given owing to reduced survival of transfused platelets, but may be used in conjunction with the treatments discussed earlier in situations of life-threatening bleeding or after head trauma[30,31]; this is in contrast with thrombotic thrombocytopenic purpura (TTP), atypical hemolytic uremic syndrome (aHUS), and HIT, in which platelet transfusions are contraindicated because of concerns of disease exacerbation and increased risk of arterial thrombosis and mortality.[31,32] For patients who fail first-line therapy, second-line treatments include splenectomy, rituximab, or the thrombopoietin receptor agonists eltrombopag or romiplostim.[23,33]

Case 2

Suppose the patient discussed earlier had the same presentation but without an antecedent upper respiratory infection, and instead with a history of recent alcohol intake. What would be an important question to ask to better define the cause of his thrombocytopenia?

Isolated thrombocytopenia without systemic symptoms in the setting of a recent ingestion raises suspicion for DITP. The thrombocytopenia in DITP usually occurs within 5 to 7 days of drug exposure and is often profound, with a platelet count less than 10×10^9/L to 20×10^9/L. A variety of mechanisms underlie the pathogenesis of DITP, the unifying concept being the development of antibodies directed against platelet epitopes that bind strongly only in the presence of a sensitizing agent.[34] Medications commonly associated with DITP include penicillins, cephalosporins, vancomycin, sulfonamide antibiotics, quinine, nonsteroidal antiinflammatory drugs, eptifibatide, abciximab, phenytoin, and valproic acid[35,36]; a more comprehensive list of suspected agents is available from the University of Oklahoma (http://www.ouhsc.edu/platelets).[34] Cessation of the offending agent is the mainstay of treatment of DITP, with platelet counts usually recovering by 1 week later.[35] Drug-dependent antibody testing in suspected cases of DITP is performed by the Blood Center of Wisconsin and can be useful to establish the diagnosis (https://www.bcw.edu/bcw/index.htm).

Historically, quinine was one of the most common causes of DITP.[37] Although no longer widely available, it is still used for relief of muscle cramps and is found in tonic water.[38,39] In the patient presented here, inquiry into the types of alcoholic beverages ingested would be useful, because a predilection for gin and tonic might suggest quinine as the cause of DITP.

Case 3

A 43-year-old woman with metastatic thyroid cancer develops shortness of breath and left lower extremity swelling and is diagnosed with bilateral pulmonary emboli (PE) and deep vein thrombosis (DVT) of the proximal left leg. She is anticoagulated with intravenous unfractionated heparin (UFH), then transitioned to low-molecular-weight heparin (LMWH). She received chemotherapy 3 weeks before her current presentation. Her initial platelet count at the time of diagnosis of PE and DVT is 150×10^9/L; 5 days after starting anticoagulation she develops progressive thrombocytopenia with a nadir of 50×10^9/L. What is the cause of her thrombocytopenia?

A broad differential for this patient's thrombocytopenia includes factors related to her cancer (eg, therapy-induced bone marrow suppression, TTP caused by chemotherapy or by cancer, direct involvement of the bone marrow or spleen by tumor, or DIC[40]), platelet consumption caused by her extensive thrombotic burden, infection, or medications such as UFH or LMWH. The timing and severity of thrombocytopenia in relation to heparin exposure are concerning for HIT.

HIT is an immune-mediated disorder characterized by production of immunoglobulin (Ig) G antibodies with specificity against complexes of platelet factor 4 (PF4, a component of platelet alpha granules) and heparin.[41,42] The large complexes of HIT antibody, PF4, and heparin then bind to and activate platelets, causing release of procoagulant substances and an increased risk of venous and arterial thrombosis.[43,44] The reported incidence of HIT ranges from 0.5% to 5% in adults treated with UFH, versus 0.2% with LMWH.[45] Treatment of HIT involves cessation of all heparin products and initiation of a nonheparin anticoagulant.[46]

Laboratory testing for HIT consists of screening tests and confirmatory tests. The major screening test is an enzyme-linked immunosorbent assay (EIA) that identifies anti-PF4/heparin IgG, IgM, and IgA antibodies.[47] The EIA has rapid turnaround time and good sensitivity and negative predictive value but poor specificity,[44,47] because false-positive tests can occur in antiphospholipid antibody syndrome, lupus, or following cardiac or orthopedic surgery.[47–49] A positive heparin-PF4 EIA must be followed by a confirmatory functional assay, the most common of which is the serotonin release assay (SRA), which measures platelet activation and degranulation in the presence of heparin.[46] Although highly specific for HIT, the SRA is a technically challenging, time-consuming assay and is performed only at certain reference laboratories.[47]

HIT is a clinicopathologic diagnosis requiring a characteristic clinical picture and identification of PF4/heparin antibodies by both screening and functional assays.[47] It also is a medical emergency, and, in the acute setting, rapid decisions must often be made about anticoagulation before return of laboratory test results.[13] The 4 Ts score (**Table 2**) is a tool designed to help clinicians predict the probability of HIT[50] and carries a high negative predictive value.[51] The HIT expert probability score consists of 8 variables identified by 26 experts on HIT, although studies thus far suggest a similar performance to the 4 Ts score.[52,53] Current treatment algorithms recommend

Table 2
The 4Ts score for pretest probability of HIT

	0 Point	1 Point	2 Points
Thrombocytopenia	Platelet count decrease <30% or platelet nadir <10 × 10⁹/L	Platelet count decrease 30%–50% or platelet nadir 10–20 × 10⁹/L	Platelet count decrease >50% or platelet nadir ≥20 × 10⁹/L
Timing of platelet decrease	Platelet count decrease <4 d without recent heparin exposure	Platelet count decrease days 5–10 (but not clear), or decrease after day 10, or decrease ≤1 d and heparin exposure within the past 30–100 d	Clear onset of platelet count decrease between days 5–10 or platelet count decrease ≤1 d with heparin exposure within the past 30 d
Thrombosis	None	Progressive or recurrent thrombosis, nonnecrotizing skin lesions, suspected but unproven thrombosis	New thrombosis, skin necrosis at sites of heparin injection, or acute systemic reaction after intravenous heparin bolus
Other causes of thrombocytopenia	Definite	Possible	None apparent

Low pretest probability, 0 to 3; intermediate pretest probability, 4 to 5; high pretest probability, 6 to 8.

Adapted from Cuker A. Clinical and laboratory diagnosis of heparin-induced thrombocytopenia: an integrated approach. Semin Thromb Hemost 2014;40(1):106–14; and Lo GK, Juhl D, Warkentin TE, et al. Evaluation of pretest clinical score (4 T's) for the diagnosis of heparin-induced thrombocytopenia in two clinical settings. J Thromb Haemost 2006;4(4):760.

stopping heparin and pursuing HIT laboratory testing only in patients with intermediate and high 4 Ts scores of greater than or equal to 4.[46]

This patient has a 4 Ts score of 5, consistent with an intermediate probability of HIT. Her anticoagulation is changed to argatroban. EIA and SRA later return positive, confirming a diagnosis of HIT. Her platelet count normalizes over the next several days. Warfarin is added, with continuation of argatroban as bridging therapy. Per institutional protocol, the two anticoagulants are continued simultaneously for 5 days; an INR on the fifth day of bridging is more than 4, at which point argatroban is stopped, and a repeat INR is measured 4 hours later and found to be 2.2. Argatroban is then stopped and warfarin continued.

Options for acute anticoagulation in HIT include a direct thrombin inhibitor (DTI) such as argatroban, bivalirudin, lepirudin, or the factor Xa inhibitor danaparoid; fondaparinux is also used off label, although cases of fondaparinux-induced HIT have been reported.[46,54,55] Direct oral anticoagulants are not recommended, although a recent, small phase II trial of rivaroxaban in HIT reported encouraging outcomes.[56] Parenteral anticoagulation must be continued as monotherapy until the platelet count recovers to the normal range before warfarin is added because of the risk of warfarin-induced protein C deficiency, which may worsen clot burden and cause limb gangrene in acute HIT.[46,57] Once warfarin is started, there should be at least a 5-day overlap with the DTI or factor Xa inhibitor, with attainment of a therapeutic INR before parenteral anticoagulation is stopped.[46,54] Patients with HIT and thrombosis are treated with 3 to 6 months of anticoagulation. The optimal duration of anticoagulation in patients with HIT without thrombosis is unclear; current recommendations suggest 4 weeks or at least until stable platelet recovery.[46,54]

Case 4

A previously healthy 34-year-old woman presents with left facial numbness, headache, and bruising over the past 3 weeks. She denies diarrhea. Her blood pressure is 100/60 mm Hg. Laboratory studies show a WBC count of 8.2 × 1000/μL, hemoglobin level 9.5 g/dL, platelet count 20 × 10⁹/L, creatinine level 1.5 mg/dL, lactate dehydrogenase level (LDH) 1330 U/L (normal, 118–242 U/L), haptoglobin level less than 10 mg/dL (normal, 30–200 mg/dL), and normal PT, PTT, and INR. Peripheral blood smear is shown in **Fig. 3**. What is this patient's diagnosis, and how should she be managed?

The combination of anemia, schistocytes, thrombocytopenia, and organ injury raises concern for a thrombotic microangiopathy (TMA).[58] The presence of greater than 1% schistocytes on peripheral blood smear with microangiopathic hemolytic anemia (MAHA) defines TMA.[58,59] Conditions associated with TMA include TTP, congenital TTP (Upshaw-Shulman syndrome), classic HUS caused by Shiga toxin–producing *Escherichia coli* hemolytic uremic syndrome (STEC-HUS), aHUS, drug-induced TMA, DIC, catastrophic antiphospholipid antibody syndrome, malignant hypertension, preeclampsia, hemolysis, elevated liver enzymes, low platelets (HELLP) syndrome, cocaine use, metastatic cancer, and scleroderma crisis.[60,61] In each of these disorders, microvascular damage leads to platelet activation and aggregation with subsequent thrombosis, thrombocytopenia, and ischemia-induced organ injury; the schistocytes arise from red blood cells traveling through vessels partially occluded by platelets.

The identification of 2 or more schistocytes per 100-times high-powered field on peripheral blood smear in the context of MAHA can satisfy a picture of TMA. However, in the 3 major TMA disorders of TTP, STEC-HUS, and aHUS, many more schistocytes are typically seen. In the past, TTP was associated with neurologic symptoms, aHUS with renal injury, and STEC-HUS in children with bloody diarrhea,[62] but there

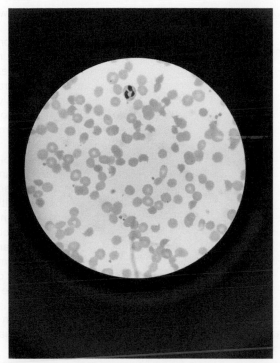

Fig. 3. Peripheral blood smear for case 3. Thrombocytopenia and multiple schistocytes are seen, suggestive of thrombotic microangiopathy (hematoxylin-eosin, original magnification ×100).

is considerable overlap in clinical presentation of these 3 conditions. Patients presenting with unexplained TMA are often initially assumed to have TTP and are treated as such until additional diagnostic results return.

TTP is caused by either congenital or acquired (via production of autoimmune inhibitors) deficiency of the von Willebrand factor (vWF) cleaving protease, ADAMTS13 **(Fig. 4)**.[63,64] The normal function of ADAMTS13 is to cleave large multimers of vWF; when ADAMTS13 is deficient or absent, platelets adhere to the resultant ultralarge vWF multimers anchored to endothelial cells, forming platelet thrombi throughout the microvasculature.[58] Thrombocytopenia, MAHA, renal failure, neurologic deficits, and fever comprise the classic pentad of TTP, but only about 5% of patients show all of these symptoms. Other common presenting complaints include nausea, vomiting, abdominal pain, diarrhea, confusion, headache, general weakness, and bleeding.[65,66]

A low ADAMTS13 level of less than 10% supports a picture of TTP rather than the other TMA disorders. Historically this test has not offered sufficient sensitivity, specificity, or turnaround time to guide acute treatment decisions, although many institutions now have in-house ADAMTS13 assays with rapid turnaround time.[67–69] At present, the initial diagnosis of TTP remains largely clinical.

TTP is a hematologic emergency with a mortality of 90% if left untreated.[68] Frontline treatment is plasma exchange (PEX), which replaces the deficient ADAMTS13 and removes anti-ADAMTS13 antibodies. Corticosteroids (eg, prednisone 1 mg/kg daily) are usually added to suppress ADAMTS13 inhibitor production[70]; rituximab may also have an adjunctive role in preventing disease relapse. Current recommendations

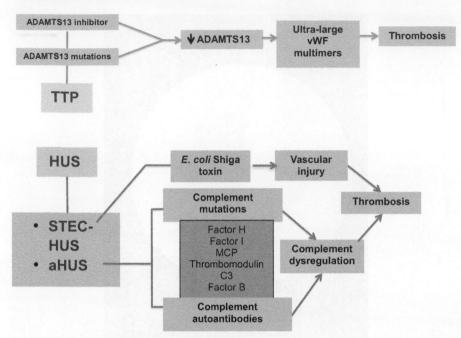

Fig. 4. Pathogenesis of TTP, STEC-HUS, and aHUS.

support initiating PEX in patients with TMA and MAHA for presumed TTP if an alternative cause has not been established.[65,70] While on PEX, complete blood counts, LDH, and blood smears are followed routinely; PEX should be continued until attainment of normal platelet counts for 2 days. Steroids can be tapered off if the platelet count remains normal for 1 to 2 weeks, at which point the plasma exchange catheter can be removed.[65]

The patient is started on prednisone 1 mg/kg. A central venous catheter is placed for initiation of daily PEX. Over the next 4 days, her platelet count increases to 70×10^9/L, but her renal function deteriorates, with an increase in creatinine level to 5 mg/dL. Pretreatment ADAMTS13 activity returns normal at 80%. Blood cultures are negative.

Poor response to PEX and a pretreatment ADAMTS13 activity of greater than 10% raise suspicion for an alternative diagnosis to TTP, such as aHUS, sepsis, malignancy, or an autoimmune disorder.[64,65,70] Although neurologic symptoms, gastrointestinal complains, and renal injury may be seen in both TTP and aHUS, severe renal involvement and progression to dialysis occur more often in aHUS.[64,71] Most cases of aHUS are caused by abnormal activation of the alternative complement pathway because of inherited or acquired mutations in genes involved in complement regulation (eg, factor H, factor I, MCP, or thrombomodulin) or in complement activation (eg, C3 or factor B) (see **Fig. 4**).[70–72] Mutation screening and identification of factor H autoantibodies can confirm a diagnosis of aHUS, but these tests are limited by lengthy turnaround time. Measurement of complement levels (eg, C3; C4; or factors H, I, or B) is done routinely but has limited utility because only about half of patients with aHUS show a reduction in C3 levels, as would be expected from alternative complement activation.[72,73]

PEX is partially effective in aHUS because it replaces missing complement factors and removes mutated components and autoantibodies.[73] Eculizumab is a monoclonal antibody against the terminal complement component C5, blocking formation of the

C5-C9 membrane attack complex and stopping further complement-mediated organ injury.[64] Eculizumab induces significant and lasting improvements in renal function, and should be started as soon as possible in patients with suspected aHUS to improve chances for renal recovery.[71,74] Because of infectious risks, patients must be vaccinated against *Neisseria meningitidis* before initiation.[75] Dosing is 900 mg intravenously (IV) weekly for 4 weeks, followed by maintenance therapy with 1200 mg IV every other week.[71,74] Patients who respond are generally kept on this agent indefinitely because of a high risk of relapse when the medication is stopped.

PEX is discontinued and eculizumab started. Over the next 14 days, her platelet count increases steadily to the range of 200 × 10^9/L, concomitant with a decrease in LDH level and improvement in creatinine level to 3.0 mg/dL. She is discharged to home with a plan for ongoing eculizumab and close outpatient follow-up. Genetic testing identifies a mutation in the complement factor H gene, the most common gene affected in aHUS.

REFERENCES

1. Kaushansky K. Thrombopoietin: the primary regulator of platelet production. Blood 1995;86(2):419–31.
2. Franco AT, Corken A, Ware J. Platelets at the interface of thrombosis, inflammation, and cancer. Blood 2015;126(5):582–8.
3. Zimmer J, Hentges F, Andres E. Borderline thrombocytopenia or mild idiopathic thrombocytopenic purpura? PLoS Med 2006;3(8):e362 [author reply: e365].
4. Stasi R, Amadori S, Osborn J, et al. Long-term outcome of otherwise healthy individuals with incidentally discovered borderline thrombocytopenia. PLoS Med 2006;3(3):e24.
5. Psaila B, Petrovic A, Page LK, et al. Intracranial hemorrhage (ICH) in children with immune thrombocytopenia (ITP): study of 40 cases. Blood 2009;114(23): 4777–83.
6. Arnold DM. Bleeding complications in immune thrombocytopenia. Hematology Am Soc Hematol Educ Program 2015;2015:237–42.
7. Izak M, Bussel JB. Management of thrombocytopenia. F1000prime Rep 2014;6: 45.
8. Crowther MA, Cook DJ, Meade MO, et al. Thrombocytopenia in medical-surgical critically ill patients: prevalence, incidence, and risk factors. J Crit Care 2005; 20(4):348–53.
9. Strauss R, Wehler M, Mehler K, et al. Thrombocytopenia in patients in the medical intensive care unit: bleeding prevalence, transfusion requirements, and outcome. Crit Care Med 2002;30(8):1765–71.
10. Vanderschueren S, De Weerdt A, Malbrain M, et al. Thrombocytopenia and prognosis in intensive care. Crit Care Med 2000;28(6):1871–6.
11. Terrell DR, Beebe LA, George JN, et al. Referral of patients with thrombocytopenia from primary care clinicians to hematologists. Blood 2009;113(17):4126–7.
12. Salib MCR, Clare R, Wang G, et al. Difficulties in establishing the cause of thrombocytopenia among ambulatory patients referred to hematology: an agreement study [abstract]. 56th American Society Annual Meeting. San Francisco CA, December, 2014. [abstract 3521].
13. Stasi R. How to approach thrombocytopenia. Hematology Am Soc Hematol Educ Program 2012;2012:191–7.
14. McMillan R. Chronic idiopathic thrombocytopenic purpura. N Engl J Med 1981; 304(19):1135–47.

15. Cooper N, Bussel J. The pathogenesis of immune thrombocytopaenic purpura. Br J Haematol 2006;133(4):364–74.

16. Hou M, Stockelberg D, Kutti J, et al. Antibodies against platelet GPIb/IX, GPIIb/IIIa, and other platelet antigens in chronic idiopathic thrombocytopenic purpura. Eur J Haematol 1995;55(5):307–14.

17. Najaoui A, Bakchoul T, Stoy J, et al. Autoantibody-mediated complement activation on platelets is a common finding in patients with immune thrombocytopenic purpura (ITP). Eur J Haematol 2012;88(2):167–74.

18. Mahabir VK, Ross C, Popovic S, et al. A blinded study of bone marrow examinations in patients with primary immune thrombocytopenia. Eur J Haematol 2013; 90(2):121–6.

19. Rodeghiero F, Stasi R, Gernsheimer T, et al. Standardization of terminology, definitions and outcome criteria in immune thrombocytopenic purpura of adults and children: report from an international working group. Blood 2009;113(11): 2386–93.

20. Bussel JB. Therapeutic approaches to secondary immune thrombocytopenic purpura. Semin Hematol 2009;46(1 Suppl 2):S44–58.

21. Neylon AJ, Saunders PW, Howard MR, et al. Clinically significant newly presenting autoimmune thrombocytopenic purpura in adults: a prospective study of a population-based cohort of 245 patients. Br J Haematol 2003;122(6):966–74.

22. Norgaard M, Cetin K, Maegbaek ML, et al. Risk of arterial thrombotic and venous thromboembolic events in patients with primary chronic immune thrombocytopenia: a Scandinavian population-based cohort study. Br J Haematol 2015;174: 639–42.

23. Provan D, Stasi R, Newland AC, et al. International consensus report on the investigation and management of primary immune thrombocytopenia. Blood 2010; 115(2):168–86.

24. Michel M, Chanet V, Dechartres A, et al. The spectrum of Evans syndrome in adults: new insight into the disease based on the analysis of 68 cases. Blood 2009;114(15):3167–72.

25. Cines DB, Bussel JB, Liebman HA, et al. The ITP syndrome: pathogenic and clinical diversity. Blood 2009;113(26):6511–21.

26. Stasi R, Sarpatwari A, Segal JB, et al. Effects of eradication of Helicobacter pylori infection in patients with immune thrombocytopenic purpura: a systematic review. Blood 2009;113(6):1231–40.

27. Scaradavou A, Bussel J. Evans syndrome. Results of a pilot study utilizing a multiagent treatment protocol. J Pediatr Hematol Oncol 1995;17(4):290–5.

28. Neunert C, Lim W, Crowther M, et al. The American Society of Hematology 2011 evidence-based practice guideline for immune thrombocytopenia. Blood 2011; 117(16):4190–207.

29. Wei Y, Ji XB, Wang YW, et al. High-dose dexamethasone vs prednisone for treatment of adult immune thrombocytopenia: a prospective multicenter randomized trial. Blood 2016;127(3):296–302.

30. Cines DB, Bussel JB. How I treat idiopathic thrombocytopenic purpura (ITP). Blood 2005;106(7):2244–51.

31. British Committee for Standards in Haematology, Blood Transfusion Task Force. Guidelines for the use of platelet transfusions. Br J Haematol 2003;122(1):10–23.

32. Goel R, Ness PM, Takemoto CM, et al. Platelet transfusions in platelet consumptive disorders are associated with arterial thrombosis and in-hospital mortality. Blood 2015;125(9):1470–6.

33. Ghanima W, Godeau B, Cines DB, et al. How I treat immune thrombocytopenia: the choice between splenectomy or a medical therapy as a second-line treatment. Blood 2012;120(5):960–9.
34. George JN, Aster RH. Drug-induced thrombocytopenia: pathogenesis, evaluation, and management. Hematology Am Soc Hematol Educ Program 2009;153–8.
35. Aster RH, Bougie DW. Drug-induced immune thrombocytopenia. N Engl J Med 2007;357(6):580–7.
36. Reese JA, Li X, Hauben M, et al. Identifying drugs that cause acute thrombocytopenia: an analysis using 3 distinct methods. Blood 2010;116(12):2127–33.
37. George JN, Raskob GE, Shah SR, et al. Drug-induced thrombocytopenia: a systematic review of published case reports. Ann Intern Med 1998;129(11):886–90.
38. Cavalli G, Guglielmi B, Ponzoni M, et al. A bitter effect: thrombocytopenia induced by a quinidine-containing beverage. Am J Med 2014;127(8):e1–2.
39. Mohamed M, Hayes R. Quinine-induced severe thrombocytopenia: the importance of taking a detailed drug history. BMJ Case Rep 2013;2013:1–2.
40. Liebman HA. Thrombocytopenia in cancer patients. Thromb Res 2014;133(Suppl 2):S63–9.
41. Amiral J, Bridey F, Dreyfus M, et al. Platelet factor 4 complexed to heparin is the target for antibodies generated in heparin-induced thrombocytopenia. Thromb Haemost 1992;68(1):95–6.
42. Kelton JG, Smith JW, Warkentin TE, et al. Immunoglobulin G from patients with heparin-induced thrombocytopenia binds to a complex of heparin and platelet factor 4. Blood 1994;83(11):3232–9.
43. Kelton JG, Warkentin TE. Heparin-induced thrombocytopenia: a historical perspective. Blood 2008;112(7):2607–16.
44. Warkentin TE. New approaches to the diagnosis of heparin-induced thrombocytopenia. Chest 2005;127(2 Suppl):35S–45S.
45. Martel N, Lee J, Wells PS. Risk for heparin-induced thrombocytopenia with unfractionated and low-molecular-weight heparin thromboprophylaxis: a meta-analysis. Blood 2005;106(8):2710–5.
46. Cuker A, Cines DB. How I treat heparin-induced thrombocytopenia. Blood 2012; 119(10):2209–18.
47. Cuker A. Clinical and laboratory diagnosis of heparin-induced thrombocytopenia: an integrated approach. Semin Thromb Hemost 2014;40(1):106–14.
48. Pauzner R, Greinacher A, Selleng K, et al. False-positive tests for heparin-induced thrombocytopenia in patients with antiphospholipid syndrome and systemic lupus erythematosus. J Thromb Haemost 2009;7(7):1070–4.
49. Bito S, Miyata S, Migita K, et al. Mechanical prophylaxis is a heparin-independent risk for anti-platelet factor 4/heparin antibody formation after orthopedic surgery. Blood 2015;127:1036–43.
50. Lo GK, Juhl D, Warkentin TE, et al. Evaluation of pretest clinical score (4 T's) for the diagnosis of heparin-induced thrombocytopenia in two clinical settings. J Thromb Haemost 2006;4(4):759–65.
51. Cuker A, Gimotty PA, Crowther MA, et al. Predictive value of the 4Ts scoring system for heparin-induced thrombocytopenia: a systematic review and meta-analysis. Blood 2012;120(20):4160–7.
52. Cuker A, Arepally G, Crowther MA, et al. The HIT Expert Probability (HEP) score: a novel pre-test probability model for heparin-induced thrombocytopenia based on broad expert opinion. J Thromb Haemost 2010;8(12):2642–50.
53. Joseph L, Gomes MP, Al Solaiman F, et al. External validation of the HIT Expert Probability (HEP) score. Thromb Haemost 2015;113(3):633–40.

54. Linkins LA, Dans AL, Moores LK, et al. Treatment and prevention of heparin-induced thrombocytopenia: antithrombotic therapy and prevention of thrombosis, 9th ed: American College of Chest Physicians Evidence-Based Clinical Practice Guidelines. Chest 2012;141(2 Suppl):e495S–530S.

55. Warkentin TE, Maurer BT, Aster RH. Heparin-induced thrombocytopenia associated with fondaparinux. N Engl J Med 2007;356(25):2653–5 [discussion: 2653–5].

56. Linkins LA WT, Pai M, Shivakumar S, et al. Rivaroxaban for treatment of suspected or confirmed heparin-induced thrombocytopenia study [Abstract]. 57th American Society Annual Meeting, Orlando, FL, December, 2015.

57. Warkentin TE, Elavathil LJ, Hayward CP, et al. The pathogenesis of venous limb gangrene associated with heparin-induced thrombocytopenia. Ann Intern Med 1997;127(9):804–12.

58. Moake JL. Thrombotic microangiopathies. N Engl J Med 2002;347(8):589–600.

59. Zini G, d'Onofrio G, Briggs C, et al. ICSH recommendations for identification, diagnostic value, and quantitation of schistocytes. Int J Lab Hematol 2012; 34(2):107–16.

60. Al-Nouri ZL, Reese JA, Terrell DR, et al. Drug-induced thrombotic microangiopathy: a systematic review of published reports. Blood 2015;125(4):616–8.

61. George JN, Nester CM. Syndromes of thrombotic microangiopathy. N Engl J Med 2014;371(19):1847–8.

62. Tarr PI, Gordon CA, Chandler WL. Shiga-toxin-producing *Escherichia coli* and haemolytic uraemic syndrome. Lancet 2005;365(9464):1073–86.

63. Furlan M, Robles R, Galbusera M, et al. von Willebrand factor-cleaving protease in thrombotic thrombocytopenic purpura and the hemolytic-uremic syndrome. N Engl J Med 1998;339(22):1578–84.

64. Tsai HM. Autoimmune thrombotic microangiopathy: advances in pathogenesis, diagnosis, and management. Semin Thromb Hemost 2012;38(5):469–82.

65. George JN. How I treat patients with thrombotic thrombocytopenic purpura: 2010. Blood 2010;116(20):4060–9.

66. Vesely SK, George JN, Lammle B, et al. ADAMTS13 activity in thrombotic thrombocytopenic purpura-hemolytic uremic syndrome: relation to presenting features and clinical outcomes in a prospective cohort of 142 patients. Blood 2003;102(1): 60–8.

67. George JN, Al-Nouri ZL. Diagnostic and therapeutic challenges in the thrombotic thrombocytopenic purpura and hemolytic uremic syndromes. Hematology Am Soc Hematol Educ Program 2012;2012:604–9.

68. Sayani FA, Abrams CS. How I treat refractory thrombotic thrombocytopenic purpura. Blood 2015;125(25):3860–7.

69. Sadler JE. Von Willebrand factor, ADAMTS13, and thrombotic thrombocytopenic purpura. Blood 2008;112(1):11–8.

70. Scully M, Goodship T. How I treat thrombotic thrombocytopenic purpura and atypical haemolytic uraemic syndrome. Br J Haematol 2014;164(6):759–66.

71. Cataland SR, Wu HM. How I treat: the clinical differentiation and initial treatment of adult patients with atypical hemolytic uremic syndrome. Blood 2014;123(16): 2478–84.

72. Nester CM, Thomas CP. Atypical hemolytic uremic syndrome: what is it, how is it diagnosed, and how is it treated? Hematology Am Soc Hematol Educ Program 2012;2012:617–25.

73. Noris M, Remuzzi G. Genetics and genetic testing in hemolytic uremic syndrome/ thrombotic thrombocytopenic purpura. Semin Nephrol 2010;30(4):395–408.

74. Legendre CM, Licht C, Muus P, et al. Terminal complement inhibitor eculizumab in atypical hemolytic-uremic syndrome. N Engl J Med 2013;368(23):2169–81.
75. Struijk GH, Bouts AH, Rijkers GT, et al. Meningococcal sepsis complicating eculizumab treatment despite prior vaccination. Am J Transplant 2013;13(3):819–20.

Novel Developments in Leukopenia and Pancytopenia

 CrossMark

Chisom Onuoha, MD[a], Junaid Arshad, MD[a], John Astle, MD, PhD[b,c],
Mina Xu, MD[b], Stephanie Halene, MD[d],*

KEYWORDS

- Leukopenia • Neutropenia • Pancytopenia • Clonal hematopoiesis
- Hemophagocytosis • Aleukemic leukemia • Large granular lymphocytosis

KEY POINTS

- Pancytopenia and leukopenia are caused by several hematopoiesis intrinsic and extrinsic processes; their duration and the company they keep (white blood cell differential, mean corpuscular volume, red cell distribution width, reticulocyte count, mean platelet volume, liver function tests) can shed light on their cause.
- A careful history and examination and review of medications are essential in determining the first steps to be taken.
- Severity of the cytopenias and concurrent symptoms determine acute management, and whenever in doubt consult a hematologist.
- Inherited disorders of childhood, such as the bone marrow failure disorders and familial hemophagocytic lymphohistiocytosis, provide mechanistic insights into acquired disorders in the adult.
- The 2 life-threatening causes of pancytopenia, acute promyelocytic leukemia (APL) and hemophagocytic lymphohistiocytosis (HLH), should be suspected in patients with fever, bleeding or bruising, and fatigue (APL) or fever, malaise, splenomegaly, hyperferritinemia, altered mental status, with or without a possible underlying rheumatologic disease (HLH).

INTRODUCTION

Cytopenias are generally discovered during investigation for causes of abnormal clinical findings, such as fatigue, bleeding, or fever, or incidentally when blood is drawn for routine checkups or other reasons. Cytopenias are not a disease entity in and of

Disclosure: The authors declare no relevant conflict of interest.
[a] Department of Medicine, St. Mary's Hospital, Waterbury, CT, USA; [b] Department of Pathology, Yale University School of Medicine, New Haven, CT, USA; [c] Department of Pathology and Laboratory Medicine, Hospital of the University of Pennsylvania, Philadelphia, PA, USA; [d] Section of Hematology, Department of Internal Medicine, Yale Comprehensive Cancer Center, Yale University School of Medicine, 300 George Street, 786E, New Haven, CT 06511, USA
* Corresponding author.
E-mail address: Stephanie.halene@yale.edu

themselves; rather, they are the expression of various underlying disease processes and may even be normal, as in the case of ethnic neutropenia. Pancytopenia is defined as the simultaneous presence of anemia, leukopenia, and thrombocytopenia on complete blood count. The parameters that define the cytopenias are given in **Table 1**.

The differential diagnosis for the causes of cytopenias is very broad. Thus, rather than going into depth for each disease, the authors here seek to provide the clinician with an approach toward identifying the underlying cause and first steps in their management. The authors concisely discuss a few causes of pancytopenia and isolated leukopenias while referring the reader to other articles in this issue for detailed discussions on isolated anemia, thrombocytopenia, leukemia, lymphoma, and plasma cell dyscrasia, each of which can cause cytopenias.

CAUSE

The processes that cause cytopenias are hematopoiesis intrinsic or extrinsic. Hematopoiesis intrinsic processes arise in hematopoietic stem or progenitor cells, such as in bone marrow failure syndromes, myelodysplasia (MDS), leukemia, lymphoma, and others. Hematopoiesis extrinsic processes include destructive processes, such as autoimmune processes, immune dysfunction such as hemophagocytic lymphohistiocytosis, hypersplenism due to liver disease, and others. These processes may primarily affect the bone marrow or may affect mature cells in the periphery with a compensatory response in the bone marrow. The bone marrow is a highly proliferative organ and generates more than 10^{11} red cells, platelets, and neutrophils every day. All cells arise from the hematopoietic stem cell (HSC), a rare, multipotent cell that resides in the bone marrow stem cell niche. HSCs have the unique ability to self-renew. HSCs give rise to one progenitor cell and one stem cell with each cell division, thereby maintaining hematopoiesis for the life span of the individual. The hematopoietic progenitors commit to either myeloid differentiation (ultimately giving rise to erythrocytes, megakaryocytes, granulocytes, and monocytes) or lymphoid differentiation (ultimately giving rise to B cells, T cells, or natural killer [NK] cells).[1] Hematopoiesis is highly regulated, and hematopoietic stem and progenitor cells depend on the complex bone marrow microenvironment that is intricately woven by mesenchymal stromal cells, macrophages, fat cells, endosteal cells, endothelial cells, and the sympathetic nervous system.[2,3]

Table 1 World Health Organization's criteria for cytopenia			
Category	HB g/dL	ANC × 10⁹/L	Platelets × 10⁹/L
Normal	$\geq$12 (f), $\geq$13 (m)	$\geq$1.8	$\geq$150
Cytopenic	<12 (f), <13 (m)	<1.8[a]	<150
MDS	<10	<1.8	<150
ICUS (1)	<11	<1.5	150

Abbreviations: ANC, absolute neutrophil count; f, female; HB, hemoglobin; ICUS, idiopathic cytopenias of unknown significance; m, male; MDS, myelodysplasia.
[a] In the white population, absolute neutrophil count values are higher than in people of African descent. See ethnic neutropenia.
Adapted from Valent P. Low blood counts: immune mediated, idiopathic, or myelodysplasia. Hematology Am Soc Hematol Educ Program 2012;2012:485–91.

There are multiple areas of overlap in the cause of pancytopenia and leukopenia. Cytopenias may be broadly classified as inherited or acquired (**Fig. 1**). Acquired cytopenias may be transient or chronic. Transient cytopenias are frequently attributable to medications, supplements, or infections and resolve when these are eliminated. Severe and chronic cytopenias associated with any alarming findings require medical attention and often extensive workup to identify and treat the underlying cause. The inherited disorders, in particular the bone marrow failure disorders, frequently come to attention during childhood but may rarely first present in the young adult. Over the past years, it has also become evident that genetic aberrations identified in patients with inherited disorders inform us of similar mechanisms and pathways occurring in acquired diseases in the adult highlighting common mechanisms. This finding has led to the development of targeted therapies that now in turn provide novel treatment avenues for the inherited disorders in children. Although a detailed discussion of the inherited disorders is beyond the scope of this review, a short summary of clinical findings and the underlying genetic causes will set the stage for discussion of the acquired disorders and help the practicing physician know when to suspect these disorders in young adults and refer the patients to specialists in the field.

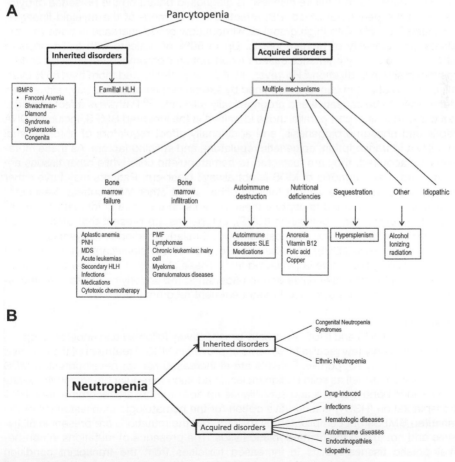

Fig. 1. (*A*) Mechanisms of pancytopenia. (*B*) Mechanisms of neutropenia.

PANCYTOPENIA
Inherited Bone Marrow Failure Syndromes and Myelodysplasia

Cause

The inherited bone marrow failure syndromes (BMFSs) are a heterogeneous group of disorders that includes Fanconi anemia (FA) (**Fig. 2**), Shwachman-Diamond syndrome (SBDS), and dyskeratosis congenita (DKC). They are caused by genetic mutations inherited from the parents or acquired de novo during intrauterine life. As these mutations are present in all cells of the body, children present not only with cytopenias but also with additional clinical findings due to the critical functions of mutated genes in several organs. Pathways affected include DNA repair (FA), ribosome maturation (SBDS), and telomere maintenance (DKC). Clinical presentations are characterized by pancytopenia and among others skin (FA, DKC), gastrointestinal (FA, SBDS), developmental, skeletal, neural, and genitourinary (FA, SBDS, DKC) abnormalities. Clinical presentations and causes of these disorders are summarized in **Table 2** and reviewed in depth in references.[4–7] The improvement and affordability of whole exome and genome sequencing over the past 10 years has not only led to identification of germline mutations underlying inherited disorders but also significantly advanced our understanding of acquired mutations resulting in hematologic diseases. MDS, an acquired bone marrow failure disorder, is diagnosed based on the presence of cytopenias in the peripheral blood (PB) affecting one or more of the myeloid lineages, dysplasia (**Fig. 3**D) with (high grade) or without (low grade) increase in bone marrow blasts, and clonality of hematopoiesis. Up to 50% of patients with a diagnosis of MDS have normal cytogenetics based on conventional chromosomal analysis or fluorescent in situ hybridization.[8] However, all of those patients, and more than 85% overall, carry mutations in genes, determined by exome sequencing, that have since been determined to be causative and prognostically relevant.[9,10] Pathways affected by genetic aberrations in part parallel those identified in the inherited BMFS, including DNA repair and ribosome biogenesis, and additionally affect regulators of chromosomal stability and transcription, epigenetic regulators, and splicing factors. As these mutations are acquired, they are restricted to hematopoietic cells while other tissues are unaffected. The diagnosis of MDS is not always clear-cut. Patients may have either cytopenias or dysplasia without fulfilling either of the other MDS criteria. New categories have been named to capture these patients. In the case of idiopathic cytopenias of undetermined significance (ICUS), cytopenias are present that otherwise do not fulfill the criteria for the diagnosis of MDS. Similarly, in idiopathic dysplasia of unknown significance (IDUS), dysplasia is present without significant cytopenias and without fulfilling MDS criteria (reviewed in[11]). These classifications allow the systematic study of the disease course and to understand the underlying cause, with the ultimate goal to provide evidence-based treatment recommendations.

Treatment

Patients with ICUS and IDUS are mostly prospectively followed and undergo supportive care, and only few receive treatments approved in MDS. Treatment of the inherited BMFSs is mostly supportive. Patients are at increased risk for development of MDS and leukemia as well as solid malignancies. In addition to regular blood counts, yearly surveillance bone marrows and surveillance for solid tumors are recommended. HSC transplantation (HSCT) is a curative option for the hematologic manifestations of the inherited BMFSs but complicated by the fact that the mutations are present in all tissues and not just in the hematopoietic tissue. The presence of mutations in non-hematopoietic tissues results in increased toxicities from the transplant condition regimen and lifelong risk of cancer and other side effects (reviewed in[4]). Management

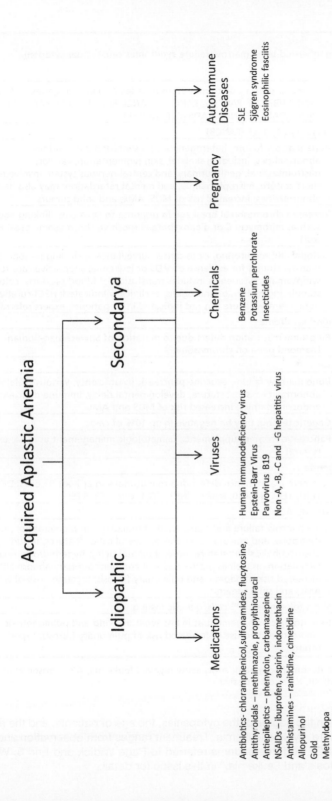

Fig. 2. Cause of aplastic anemia. [a] List not exhaustive.

Table 2
The most common inherited bone marrow failure syndromes causing pancytopenia

FA

Pathway	DNA repair defect due to mutations in at least 15 known genes: FANCA-C, FANCD1/BRCA2, FANCD2, FANCE-G, FANCI, FANCJ/BR1P1, FANCL-M, FANCN/PALB2, FANCO/RAD51C, FANCP/SLX4
Inheritance	Majority AR, 1 XR (FANCB)
Clinical	Bone marrow failure; heterogeneous presentation with various abnormalities, including skeletal, skin pigmentation, cardiac, gastrointestinal, genitourinary, and central nervous system involvement; short stature, microphthalmia, and mental retardation; may also have no abnormalities; increased risk of MDS, AML, and solid tumors
Data	Increased chromosomal breakage in response to DNA cross-linking agents, such as mitomycin C or diepoxybutane (positive chromosome breakage test)
Management	Periodic CBC monitoring, close cancer surveillance, including periodic bone marrow studies for evidence of MDS or leukemia; supportive care for symptomatic cytopenias includes transfusion of blood products, colony-stimulating factors, or androgens, as clinically indicated; HSCT curative for bone marrow failure but not indicated in all patients; expert referral

Shwachman-Diamond syndrome

Pathway	Ribosome maturation defect due to mutation of Shwachman-Bodian-Diamond gene on chromosome 7
Inheritance	AR
Clinical	Bone marrow failure, exocrine pancreatic insufficiency; various skeletal abnormalities, short stature, developmental delay, immune deficiencies, endocrinopathies; increased risk of MDS and AML
Data	Genetic testing: may be negative in up 10% of cases
Management	Pancreatic enzyme supplements; hematologic management as in FA; expert referral

Dyskeratosis congenita

Pathway	Telomere maintenance defect due to mutations in at least 9 genes: DKC1, TERT, TERC, NOP10, NHP2, TINF2, CTC1, WRAP53, RTELI
Inheritance	XR, AR, AD
Clinical	Bone marrow failure and classic triad of reticular skin pigmentation, nail dystrophy, and mucosal leukoplakia; several other features, including microcephaly, short stature, developmental delay, hyperhidrosis, excess lacrimation, as well as gastrointestinal and genitourinary abnormalities; increased risk of hepatic and pulmonary fibrosis; increased risk of MDS, AML, and solid tumors
Data	Short telomeres in PB cells, genetic testing
Management	Hematologic management as in FA; avoid smoking and pulmonotoxic medications because of increased risk of pulmonary fibrosis; expert referral

Abbreviations: AD, autosomal dominant; AML, acute myeloid leukemia; AR, autosomal recessive; PB, peripheral blood; XR, X-linked recessive.
Data from Refs.[4–7]

of MDS depends on the degree of the cytopenias, the age of patients, and the risk for progression to acute myeloid leukemia. Treatment ranges from observation and supportive care to HSCT and the reader is referred to Page Widick and Eric S. Winer's article, "Leukocytosis and Leukemia," in this issue for detail.

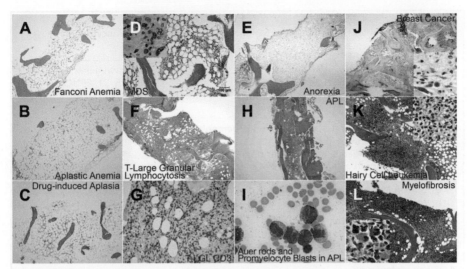

Fig. 3. Bone marrow findings in patients with pancytopenia. (*A*) Hypocellular bone marrow in a 6 year old patient with Fanconi Anemia (A, H&E, 4×). (*B*) Severely hypocellular bone marrow, Aplastic Anemia (H&E, 4×). (*C*) Drug-induced aplasia (methotrexate in setting of acute renal failure) in a 67 year old patient (H&E,4×) with rheumatoid arthritis. (*D*) Myelodysplastic marrow (H&E, 10×) with dysplastic megakaryocytes (insert, H&E 60×, oil). (*E*) Hypocellularity and gelatinous degeneration of the bone marrow in a 16 year old patient with anorexia nervosa. (*F, G*) Markedly hypercellular bone marrow in a 78 year old patient with T-Large Granular Leukemia (F, H&E, 4×) with increased T-cell infiltration (G, CD3, 20×). (*H, I*) Markedly hypercellular bone marrow in a 78 year old patient with Acute Promyelocytic Leukemia (APL) (H, H&E, 4×) with classic findings of Auer rods and abnormal promyelocytes on bone marrow aspirate (I, Wright Giemsa, 100× Oil). (*J*) Sclerotic appearing bone marrow biopsy with infiltration by non-hematopoietic cells and fibrosis in a patient with metastatic breast cancer (H&E, 4×). (*K*) Markedly hypercellular marrow (H&E, 4×) in a patient with Hairy cell leukemia with classic fried egg appearance under higher magnification (H&E, 40×). (*L*) Hypercellular marrow with fibrosis in a patient with myelofibrosis (H&E, 4×) with abnormally clustered megakaryocytes (H&E, 40×).

Familial and Acquired Hemophagocytic Lymphohistiocytosis

Although the pancytopenia in BMFSs and MDS is due to defects in the HSC, pancytopenia due to hemophagocytic lymphohistiocytosis (HLH) results from uncontrolled phagocytosis and destruction of blood cells by activated macrophages. HLH is a rare, life-threatening hyperinflammatory disorder that is rapidly fatal if treatment is delayed. As with the inherited BMFS, the underlying genetic lesions for familial HLH (FHLH) have been identified; with subclassification of FHLH into 5 genetic subtypes.[12] More than half of FHLH cases are due to mutations in the perforin gene. These cause defects in the primary cytotoxic effector pathway in lymphocytes and NK cells, thereby leading to poor clearance of target cells—particularly macrophages—and persistent immune activation.[13] FHLH predominantly manifests itself in children. In most adults, HLH is secondary to certain triggers that may or may not be superimposed on predisposing genetic backgrounds.[14,15] Unlike in FHLH, the underlying mechanisms in acquired HLH are less well understood. However, immune dysregulation with hyperinflammation due to T- and NK-cell dysfunction in the setting of malignancy, infections (viral, bacterial) (**Box 1**), underlying rheumatologic conditions, and posttransplant states seems to be the predominant process.[14–17] In the setting of

---

Box 1
Diagnostic criteria for hemophagocytic lymphohistiocytosis

1. Molecular diagnosis consistent with HLH

OR

2. Five out of the following 8 criteria:
   a. Fever
   b. Splenomegaly
   c. Cytopenias affecting 2 lineages or more: hemoglobin less than 9 g/dL, platelets less than 100,000/μL, neutrophils less than 1000/μL
   d. Hypertriglyceridemia and/or hypofibrinogenemia
   e. Hemophagocytosis in bone marrow, spleen or lymph nodes,
   f. Low or absent NK-cell activity
   g. Ferritin 500 μg/L or greater
   h. Soluble CD25 2400 U/mL or greater

Infectious triggers of acquired HLH
1. Viruses: EBV, HIV, CMV, parvovirus B19, hepatitis viruses, herpes viruses
2. Bacteria: *Mycobacterium tuberculosis*, staphylococci, rickettsiae, *Escherichia coli*
3. Parasites: *Leishmania, Plasmodium, Toxoplasma*
4. Fungi: *Histoplasma*

Abbreviations: CMV, cytomegalovirus; EBV, Epstein-Barr virus; HIV, human immunodeficiency virus.
   Data from Ramos-Casals M, Brito-Zerón P, López-Guillermo A, et al. Adult haemophagocytic syndrome. Lancet Lond Engl 2014;383(9927):1503–16; and Henter J-I, Horne A, Aricó M, et al. HLH-2004: diagnostic and therapeutic guidelines for hemophagocytic lymphohistiocytosis. Pediatr Blood Cancer 2007;48(2):124–31.

---

underlying rheumatologic disorders, in particular in systemic juvenile inflammatory arthritis, systemic lupus erythematosus (SLE), and adult-onset Still disease, HLH is called macrophage activation syndrome (MAS).

The clinical presentation of HLH is nonspecific; thus, a high index of suspicion is required to make the diagnosis. Patients can present with fever, cytopenias, and splenomegaly. Standard laboratory data reveal bicytopenia or pancytopenia, possible evidence of organ dysfunction, and disseminated intravascular coagulation (DIC) with hypofibrinogenemia. Additional testing may reveal hypertriglyceridemia. Marked hyperferritinemia prompts ordering of CD25 (soluble interleukin 2 [IL-2] receptor), which tends to also be markedly elevated, and testing of NK cell function, that may or may not be abnormal. To establish the diagnosis, 5 out 8 criteria have to be fulfilled (see **Box 1**).[18] Pancytopenia or suspicion for HLH prompts hematologic consultation and bone marrow aspiration and biopsy. Hemophagocytosis in hematopoietic tissues is one of the 8 criteria, but its presence or absence poorly predicts disease likelihood and should not sway against the diagnosis when other criteria are fulfilled.[19] As no defined criteria exist for the diagnosis of MAS, given the similarities between FHLH and MAS, use of HLH criteria facilitates the diagnosis and timely initiation of treatment.

Treatment

HLH can be rapidly fatal with greater than 50% mortality in adults. For the FHLH syndromes, treatment is well defined and proven efficacious based on the revised HLH-2004 protocol.[18] Treatment is initiated with dexamethasone/etoposide/cyclosporine in conjunction with intrathecal chemotherapy for neurologic involvement. When control of the disease is achieved, steroids are tapered with initiation of continuation therapy until HSCT. The latter is frequently the only curative approach given the inherited nature and high penetrance of the gene mutations. For acquired HLH, treatment is less standardized. Immediate treatment is aimed at controlling the overactive immune system and adapted to the clinical course and the underlying cause. Infections should be aggressively treated. In patients with rheumatologic disorders, specific treatments targeted at the underlying disorder and maintenance with agents, such as the IL-1β inhibitors, present long-term control while limiting the degree of immunosuppression. For malignancy-associated HLH/MAS, etoposide may be added to the chemotherapy regimen if appropriate. For idiopathic HLH, an etoposide-based regimen is chosen based on the HLH-2004 protocol, followed by allogeneic stem cell transplant in recurrent disease or in those without an identifiable precipitating cause (reviewed in[20]).

Aplastic Anemia

Cause

Acquired aplastic anemia (AA) is a rare disorder characterized by pancytopenia and hypocellular bone marrow without evidence of marrow fibrosis or an abnormal infiltrate (see **Figs. 2** and **3B; Table 3**). Its incidence is 1 to 3 cases per million per year, with a 2- to 3-fold higher incidence in the Far East.[21,22] The age distribution of acquired AA is bimodal with the first peak in those 10 to 25 years of age and the second peak in those more than 60 years of age with equal sex distribution.

Acquired AA is thought to be immune mediated, as evidenced by the response to immunosuppressive therapy. In most patients, a definitive cause is not established, but medications are the most commonly identified precipitants. Inherited BMFSs, hypoplastic MDS, as well as nutritional deficiencies have to be ruled out. Blast count in the bone marrow, chromosomal breakage analysis, careful analysis for dysplasia, and molecular diagnostics should be performed. Diagnostic criteria, classification, and treatment guidelines have been developed.[23]

Treatment

Any potential triggers, such as medications, should be removed. In idiopathic cases, treatment depends on severity. Observation is often appropriate for patients with nonsevere AA as long as blood counts remain stable and transfusions are not required. Patients with severe AA and very severe AA almost always require treatment.[24] Supportive therapy includes treatment of infections and transfusion of blood products as clinically

---

Table 3
Diagnostic criteria and classification of aplastic anemia

Complete Blood Count	Bone Marrow, Genetic, and PNH Testing
Any 2 of the following: • Hemoglobin <10 g/dL • Platelets <50,000 cells/μL • Neutrophils <1500 cells/μL	A hypocellular bone marrow biopsy without evidence of increased blasts or dysplasia (both of these suggest hypoplastic MDS) Absence of chromosomal aberrations and gene mutations indicating MDS or inherited BMFSs Document presence or absence of PNH clones

Assessment of severity: modified Camitta criteria
• SAA: BM cellularity <25% (or 25%–50% with <30% residual hematopoietic cells) and 2 or more of the following: (1) neutrophils <500/μL, (2) platelets <20,000/μL, and (3) reticulocyte count <20,000/μL
• VSAA: as with SAA but with neutrophil count <200/μL
• NSAA: AA not meeting criteria for SAA or VSAA

Abbreviations: NSAA, nonsevere AA; PNH, paroxysmal nocturnal hemoglobinuria; SAA, severe AA; VSAA, very severe AA.
Data from Killick SB, Bown N, Cavenagh J, et al. Guidelines for the diagnosis and management of adult aplastic anaemia. Br J Haematol 2016;172(2):187–207.

indicated; steroids are avoided because of the associated increased risk of infections. Immunosuppressive therapy (IST) with antithymocyte globulin and cyclosporine A[25,26] is the therapy of choice for a subset of patients, whereas HSCT is indicated in patients who are younger than 40 years of age with a matched sibling donor and in those who fail IST.[27] Hematopoietic growth factors, such as erythropoietin and granulocyte colony-stimulating factor, have no clear demonstrated benefits.[28] More recently, eltrombopag, a thrombopoietin receptor agonist, has been approved in the United States for treatment of patients with insufficient response to IST based on its effect not only on megakaryopoiesis but also on the HSC,[25,29] thus, increasing not only platelet counts but also other cell lines. Treatment of AA has been reviewed in detail elsewhere.[24,26]

Bone Marrow Infiltration and Myelofibrosis

Infiltration of the marrow space, also termed myelophthisis, can be associated with a variety of benign and malignant diseases. Several primary hematopoietic disorders, such as acute promyelocytic leukemia (see **Fig. 3**H, I), hairy cell leukemia (see **Fig. 3**K), large granular lymphocytosis (see **Fig. 3**F, G), multiple myeloma, and lymphoma, can involve the bone marrow and, thereby, result in pancytopenia. Of note, promyelocytic leukemia frequently presents with concurrent DIC, resulting in increased bleeding risk due to concurrent thrombocytopenia. A high level of suspicion is required for a timely diagnosis, especially if leukemic blasts are not immediately evident on PB smear (see **Fig. 3**I). Nonhematopoietic malignancies, such as breast cancer, melanoma, lung, and prostate cancer, can metastasize to the bone marrow with displacement of normal hematopoietic elements with or without concurrent fibrosis and bone remodeling (see **Fig. 3**J). In rare instances, autoimmune, metabolic, and granulomatous diseases can be associated with marrow infiltration resulting in pancytopenia. Autoimmune myelofibrosis occurs in patients with collagen vascular disorders who present with cytopenias, some mild dyspoietic changes, and mild to moderate fibrosis (occasionally with some reactive lymphoid aggregates and polyclonal plasmacytosis). This entity should be distinguished from malignant processes.[30] Pancytopenias and review of the PB smear (confirmation of the cytopenias, presence of teardrop cells, and a leukoerythroblastic picture) will call for bone marrow aspiration and biopsy and result in establishment of the diagnosis. Primary myelofibrosis (PMF) is one of the myeloproliferative disorders. Secondary myelofibrosis resulting from polycythemia vera and essential thrombocytosis is reviewed in Aric Parnes and Arvind Ravi's article, "Polycythemia and Thrombocytosis," in this issue. PMF is characterized by proliferation of myeloid cells with variable morphologic maturity and hematopoietic efficiency. Its presentation is variable and can include anemia, thrombocytopenia or thrombocytosis, and leukopenia or leukocytosis. Myelofibrosis (see **Fig. 3**L) results in extramedullary hematopoiesis with splenomegaly and occasionally hepatomegaly. Patients may present with cytopenias or with fatigue, pruritus, hepatosplenomegaly, or thrombotic events. PB smear evaluation and bone marrow biopsy are complemented by genetic analysis. Mutations in janus kinase 2, the thrombopoietin receptor MPL, or calreticulin may be present concurrent with other recurrent chromosomal aberrations and mutations identified in myeloid malignancies. Initial treatment is dictated by the risk of disease progression to leukemia and estimated overall survival as calculated by prognostic scores. PMF is also discussed in further detail (see Aric Parnes and Arvind Ravi's article, "Polycythemia and Thrombocytosis," in this issue).

Infections and Hypersplenism

Several viruses have been associated with pancytopenia, especially human immunodeficiency virus (HIV), cytomegalovirus, Epstein-Barr virus, and the hepatitis viruses.

The hematopoietic effects of HIV infection have been the subject of many studies and are thought to be a combination of viral- and medication-induced cytotoxicity to the HSC and the bone marrow microenvironment.[31] Cytopenias caused by the other viral infections are transient or resolve with treatment. Overwhelming sepsis can also cause pancytopenia that is a frequent reason for hematology consultation in the hospital. In endemic areas, *Anaplasma* and *Ehrlichia* infection can result in pancytopenia and even mimic or induce HLH. Treatment is targeted at the underlying infection accompanied by supportive care. Splenomegaly, most frequently secondary to liver cirrhosis, results in sequestration and rapid destruction of the blood cells by the reticuloendothelial system. Treatment consists of supportive care and in extreme cases of liver failure; organ transplantation will also correct cytopenias.

LEUKOPENIA
Neutropenia and Lymphopenia

Neutropenia and lymphopenia represent the main clinically significant leukopenias. The defining values are shown in **Table 1**. Acquired neutropenia is encountered relatively frequently in clinical practice. It is most often medication related, requiring discontinuation of the offending agent, due to autoimmune processes, or neoplastic, in particular MDS.

Acquired lymphopenia occurs most frequently secondary to infections (viral, bacterial) and rheumatologic disorders (SLE, rheumatoid arthritis, sarcoidosis). Advanced HIV infection is well known to cause specifically CD4+ T-cell deficiency. Treatment is tailored to the underlying cause.

Inherited conditions resulting in neutropenia and/or lymphopenia are rare but present with severe infections early in childhood. The inherited disorders include, among others, the congenital neutropenia syndromes (most notably severe congenital neutropenia and cyclic neutropenia) (reviewed in[32–34]), Wiskott-Aldrich syndrome (reviewed in[35]), and the severe combined immunodeficiency disorders (reviewed in[36]). The genetic basis for several of these disorders is known, whereas for others it is an active subject of research. Treatments are targeted at prevention and amelioration of infections. Based on the genetic background, several of these disorders, especially those affecting the lymphoid lineage, have been the subject of gene therapy trials. In addition to infections, with several of the disorders, patients are at risk for development of hematologic malignancies and cancers. HSCT is curative but carries the risk of upfront mortality and significant morbidity.

Ethnic (or constitutional) neutropenia is a distinct, benign inherited neutropenia. Affected individuals are of Yemenite Jewish, South African, West Indian, or Arab Jordanian descent and have reduced neutrophil (and lymphocyte) counts without increased susceptibility to infections. Workup including PB smear and bone marrow (BM) evaluation are normal (reviewed in[37]), and treatment is not required.

Medications

The most obvious drugs causing cytopenias are chemotherapeutic agents via direct cytotoxic effects on hematopoietic stem and progenitor cells in the bone marrow (see **Fig. 3C**).[38] Cytotoxic effects are dose related, and drug withdrawal results in gradual improvement in counts. Drugs frequently implicated in pancytopenia and/or neutropenia are certain nonsteroidal antiinflammatory drugs, antipsychotics, antiepileptics, antimicrobials, sulfonamides, and gold compounds.[39] Withdrawal of the drug may or may not result in recovery of counts. Immunosuppressive treatment, as for idiopathic aplastic anemia, may be beneficial in certain instances.

APPROACH

Diagnosis

The clinical presentation of pancytopenia or leukopenia is determined by the severity of the cytopenia and any underlying diagnosis. A careful history to determine the duration and associated symptoms and past medical, family, and social history and careful assessment of medication or supplement use and environmental exposures are the first steps. In incidentally discovered cytopenias, patients may be asymptomatic. Alternatively, patients may present with nonspecific symptoms, such as fever, fatigue, malaise, or weight loss. Localized symptoms of infection may be present; jaundice may suggest hemolysis (as in paroxysmal nocturnal hemoglobinuria) or ineffective hematopoiesis (vitamin B12 deficiency). Severe protein-calorie malnutrition encountered in patients with anorexia nervosa can result in pancytopenia with gelatinous degeneration of the bone marrow (see **Fig. 3**E). Patients with underlying autoimmune diseases, such as SLE or Sjögren syndrome, may complain of a rash, arthralgias, dry eyes, or other suggestive symptoms. A careful history of travel or exposure to travelers should be taken. Social history may reveal excessive alcohol consumption or intravenous drug use, with increased risk of hepatitis and HIV infection. Occupational history may reveal exposure to toxins (benzene was the first environmental toxin to be identified as a cause for AA) or increased risk for viral infections. The medical history and family history may suggest inherited syndromes.

A careful physical examination is of utmost necessity. Asymptomatic patients with incidentally discovered cytopenias may have no abnormal findings. On the contrary, hemodynamic instability may be present in patients with severe neutropenia and overwhelming infection, severe anemia, or in patients with HLH. Other obvious abnormalities on physical examination, such as jaundice, pallor, sinusitis, gingivitis, oral ulcers, and bleeding, may be present. The ears, lungs, heart, abdomen, skin, joints, and neurologic system should be closely examined, as findings will guide subsequent diagnostic workup.

Laboratory Examination

A routine complete blood count (CBC) with white blood cell differential, mean corpuscular volume, red cell distribution width, and mean platelet volume may give first insights into specific white cell disorders and the presence of a hypoproliferative or hyperproliferative process. With the advent of novel cell counters, reticulocyte and reticulated platelet count (elevated when new, young cells are relatively increased) may soon no longer require manual assessment and be easily available in the daily practice setting. A chemistry profile including basic metabolic and hepatic function tests, haptoglobin, lactate dehydrogenase, and iron studies including ferritin can further corroborate findings of the CBC. A PB smear evaluation is irreplaceable and can further narrow down the differential diagnosis and aid in the decision whether a specialist should be consulted and whether a bone marrow procedure is indicated. Additional investigations to exclude underlying conditions, such as antibody tests for rheumatologic diseases, viral serologies, quantitative immunoglobulins, vitamin B12, folate, and copper levels, as well as imaging (eg, computed tomography scan) may be clinically indicated. Ultimately, bone marrow aspiration and biopsy are required when a cause cannot be established from noninvasive testing or when histologic confirmation of the diagnosis is needed. Evaluation of the bone marrow aspirate smear, iron stain, flow cytometric analysis, histology of the biopsy core, and genetic studies are routine in the evaluation of bone marrow specimens. The workup of pancytopenia is summarized in **Fig. 4**.

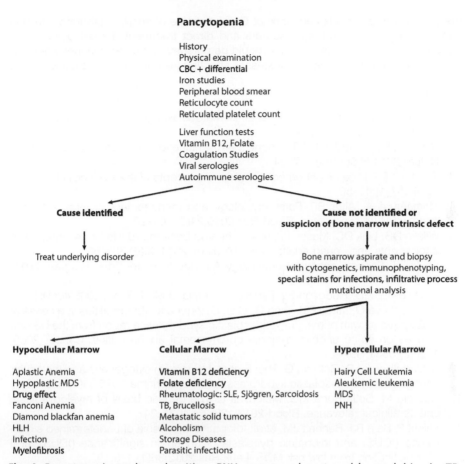

Fig. 4. Pancytopenia workup algorithm. PNH, paroxysmal nocturnal hemoglobinuria; TB, tuberculosis.

Management

For certain patients, such as those with ethnic neutropenia, no interventions are necessary and observation is sufficient. Treatment, when needed, is directed at the underlying cause. Culprit medications should be discontinued when possible. Additionally, depending on the clinical scenario, patients may also benefit from supportive therapy, such as transfusion of blood products and administration of lineage-specific stimulating growth factors, such as erythropoietin, granulocyte or granulocyte/monocyte colony-stimulating growth factor, and so-called thrombomimetics, given in place of thrombopoietin. Patients with neutropenic fever represent a hematologic/oncologic emergency, and immediate broad-spectrum antibiotic therapy and diagnostic workup are required. In cases of severe or symptomatic cytopenias, diagnostic uncertainty, rare diseases, or diseases outside the realm of general internal medicine, expert hematologist consultation should be obtained.

In summary, cytopenias are the expression of various underlying disease processes. Careful attention to details in patients' presentation, history, and examination and the ancillary parameters of the CBC with a PB smear can point the clinician toward the appropriate diagnosis and workup. Careful choice of ancillary laboratory testing can shed light on underlying disorders and direct treatment. Expert opinion and bone marrow aspiration and biopsy should be pursued in a timely manner when primary hematopoietic disorders or processes affecting the bone marrow are suspected.

REFERENCES

1. Doulatov S, Notta F, Laurenti E, et al. Hematopoiesis: a human perspective. Cell Stem Cell 2012;10(2):120–36.
2. Morrison SJ, Scadden DT. The bone marrow niche for haematopoietic stem cells. Nature 2014;505(7483):327–34.
3. Scadden DT. Nice neighborhood: emerging concepts of the stem cell niche. Cell 2014;157(1):41–50.
4. Shimamura A, Alter BP. Pathophysiology and management of inherited bone marrow failure syndromes. Blood Rev 2010;24(3):101–22.
5. Wilson DB, Link DC, Mason PJ, et al. Inherited bone marrow failure syndromes in adolescents and young adults. Annu Mediaev 2014;46(6):353–63.
6. Soulier J. Fanconi anemia. Hematology Am Soc Hematol Educ Program 2011; 2011:492–7.
7. Tischkowitz MD, Hodgson SV. Fanconi anaemia. J Med Genet 2003;40(1):1–10.
8. Pozdnyakova O, Miron PM, Tang G, et al. Cytogenetic abnormalities in a series of 1,029 patients with primary myelodysplastic syndromes: a report from the US with a focus on some undefined single chromosomal abnormalities. Cancer 2008; 113(12):3331–40.
9. Schlegelberger B, Gohring G, Thol F, et al. Update on cytogenetic and molecular changes in myelodysplastic syndromes. Leuk Lymphoma 2012;53(4):525–36.
10. Cazzola M, Della Porta MG, Malcovati L. The genetic basis of myelodysplasia and its clinical relevance. Blood 2013;122(25):4021–34.
11. Valent P, Bain BJ, Bennett JM, et al. Idiopathic cytopenia of undetermined significance (ICUS) and idiopathic dysplasia of uncertain significance (IDUS), and their distinction from low risk MDS. Leuk Res 2012;36(1):1–5.
12. Filipovich AH, Chandrakasan S. Pathogenesis of hemophagocytic lymphohistiocytosis. Hematol Oncol Clin North Am 2015;29(5):895–902.
13. Stepp SE, Dufourcq-Lagelouse R, Le Deist F, et al. Perforin gene defects in familial hemophagocytic lymphohistiocytosis. Science 1999;286(5446):1957–9.
14. Schram AM, Comstock P, Campo M, et al. Haemophagocytic lymphohistiocytosis in adults: a multicentre case series over 7 years. Br J Haematol 2016;172(3): 412–9.
15. Ramos-Casals M, Brito-Zerón P, López-Guillermo A, et al. Adult haemophagocytic syndrome. Lancet Lond Engl 2014;383(9927):1503–16.
16. Ishii E, Ohga S, Imashuku S, et al. Nationwide survey of hemophagocytic lymphohistiocytosis in Japan. Int J Hematol 2007;86(1):58–65.
17. Emmenegger U, Schach DJ, Larroche C, et al. Haemophagocytic syndromes in adults: current concepts and challenges ahead. Swiss Med Wkly 2005; 135(21–22):299–314.
18. Henter J-I, Horne A, Aricó M, et al. HLH-2004: diagnostic and therapeutic guidelines for hemophagocytic lymphohistiocytosis. Pediatr Blood Cancer 2007;48(2): 124–31.
19. Ho C, Yao X, Tian L, et al. Marrow assessment for hemophagocytic lymphohistiocytosis demonstrates poor correlation with disease probability. Am J Clin Pathol 2014;141(1):62–71.

20. Schram AM, Berliner N. How I treat hemophagocytic lymphohistiocytosis in the adult patient. Blood 2015;125(19):2908–14.
21. Mary JY, Baumelou E, Guiguet M. Epidemiology of aplastic anemia in France: a prospective multicentric study. The French Cooperative Group for Epidemiological Study of Aplastic Anemia. Blood 1990;75(8):1646–53.
22. Montané E, Ibáñez L, Vidal X, et al. Epidemiology of aplastic anemia: a prospective multicenter study. Haematologica 2008;93(4):518–23.
23. Killick SB, Bown N, Cavenagh J, et al. Guidelines for the diagnosis and management of adult aplastic anaemia. Br J Haematol 2016;172(2):187–207.
24. Scheinberg P, Young NS. How I treat acquired aplastic anemia. Blood 2012; 120(6):1185–96.
25. Olnes MJ, Scheinberg P, Calvo KR, et al. Eltrombopag and improved hematopoiesis in refractory aplastic anemia. N Engl J Med 2012;367(1):11–9.
26. Scheinberg P. Aplastic anemia: therapeutic updates in immunosuppression and transplantation. Hematology Am Soc Hematol Educ Program 2012;2012: 292–300.
27. Sureda A, Bader P, Cesaro S, et al. Indications for allo- and auto-SCT for haematological diseases, solid tumours and immune disorders: current practice in Europe, 2015. Bone Marrow Transpl 2015;50(8):1037–56.
28. DeZern AE, Brodsky RA. Clinical management of aplastic anemia. Expert Rev Hematol 2011;4(2):221–30.
29. Desmond R, Townsley DM, Dumitriu B, et al. Eltrombopag restores trilineage hematopoiesis in refractory severe aplastic anemia that can be sustained on discontinuation of drug. Blood 2014;123(12):1818–25.
30. Bass RD, Pullarkat V, Feinstein DI, et al. Pathology of autoimmune myelofibrosis. A report of three cases and a review of the literature. Am J Clin Pathol 2001; 116(2):211–6.
31. Akkina R. New insights into HIV impact on hematopoiesis. Blood 2013;122(13): 2144–6.
32. Horwitz MS, Corey SJ, Grimes HL, et al. ELANE mutations in cyclic and severe congenital neutropenia. Hematol Oncol Clin North Am 2013;27(1):19–41.
33. Dale DC, Person RE, Bolyard AA, et al. Mutations in the gene encoding neutrophil elastase in congenital and cyclic neutropenia. Blood 2000;96(7):2317–22.
34. James Ancliff P. Congenital neutropenia. Blood Rev 2003;17(4):209–16.
35. Buchbinder D, Nugent DJ, Fillipovich AH. Wiskott-Aldrich syndrome: diagnosis, current management, and emerging treatments. Appl Clin Genet 2014;7:55–66.
36. Chinn IK, Shearer WT. Severe combined immunodeficiency disorders. Immunol Allergy Clin N Am 2015;35(4):671–94.
37. Haddy TB, Rana SR, Castro O. Benign ethnic neutropenia: what is a normal absolute neutrophil count? J Lab Clin Med 1999;133(1):15–22.
38. Barreto JN, McCullough KB, Ice LL, et al. Antineoplastic agents and the associated myelosuppressive effects: a review. J Pharm Pract 2014;27(5):440–6.
39. Bhatt V, Saleem A. Drug-induced neutropenia–pathophysiology, clinical features, and management. Ann Clin Lab Sci 2004;34(2):131–7.

Leukocytosis and Leukemia

Page Widick, MD[a], Eric S. Winer, MD[b],*

KEYWORDS

- Leukocytosis • White blood cell count • Inflammation • Leukemia

KEY POINTS

- Leukocytosis may be caused by a variety of benign and malignant conditions. Careful history and laboratory evaluation can assist in differentiating these causes.
- Use of white blood cell differential as well as peripheral blood smear and morphologic characteristics may improve the ability to diagnose the underlying causative process.
- Nonmalignant causes of leukocytosis include infection, inflammation, medication, surgery, and physical/physiologic stress.
- The presence of blasts or other early progenitors of cells is highly suggestive of a primary bone marrow disorder that should prompt an immediate evaluation by a hematology specialist.
- Patients with leukemia often require chemotherapy or bone marrow transplant. Following treatment, they need to be monitored closely for late complications.

INTRODUCTION

The accepted normal range of white blood cell (WBC) counts in nonpregnant adults is approximately 4000 to 11,000 cells/mm³; thus, leukocytosis is defined as any WBC count greater than 11,000 cells/mm³ (**Table 1** for normal WBC differential). An abnormally increased leukocyte count can be caused by a wide range of benign and malignant conditions. Cell differentiation type, chronicity of abnormal values, degree of WBC increase, patient gender and ethnicity, and associated symptoms are important characteristics used to differentiate between these causes.

WHITE BLOOD CELL LINEAGES

Leukocytes are derived from 2 distinct pathways: the myeloid pathway, which produces all granulocytes and monocytes, and the lymphoid pathway, which produces

Disclosures: The authors report no commercial or financial conflicts of interest and did not receive funding for the production of this article.
a Department of Internal Medicine, Rhode Island Hospital, Brown University, JB 0100, 593 Eddy Street, Providence, RI 02903, USA; b Division of Hematology/Oncology, Rhode Island Hospital, Brown University, 593 Eddy Street, Providence, RI 02903, USA
* Corresponding author.
E-mail address: erics_winer@dfci.harvard.edu

Prim Care Clin Office Pract 43 (2016) 575–587
http://dx.doi.org/10.1016/j.pop.2016.07.007
0095-4543/16/© 2016 Elsevier Inc. All rights reserved.

Table 1
Normal leukocyte distribution in a complete blood count with differential

White Blood Cell Lines	Total Leukocyte Count (%)
Lymphocytes	20–40
Neutrophils	40–60
Monocytes	2–8
Eosinophils	1–4
Basophils	0.5–1

B and T lymphocytes. Granulocytes, including neutrophils, basophils, and eosinophils, are the major cellular components in inflammatory and antimicrobial responses. These cells are produced in the bone marrow, which stores roughly 90% of all granulocytes in the body. A small percentage of neutrophils are also present along the endothelium of blood vessels. The localization of these two granulocyte populations allows rapid upregulation of granulocyte production as well as prompt mobilization in response to external stress.[1]

Monocytes comprise another subset of the myeloid pathway, and these cells function by consuming foreign material. Monocytes are produced within the bone marrow. On traveling to damaged tissues, monocytes differentiate into tissue-fixed macrophages that are responsible for consumption of local pathogens.

In contrast with cells of the myeloid lineage, which mount a nonspecific innate immune response, the cells in the lymphoid lineage directly respond to specific antigens. B cells respond to antigens encountered in the blood, whereas T cells are activated by the presentation of antigens by other cells. The presentation of an antigen to either of these types of lymphocytes activates clonal proliferation aimed at that particular target. Proliferation of any of these cell types (neutrophils, basophils, eosinophils, monocytes, or lymphocytes) can result in a peripheral leukocytosis (**Fig. 1**); however, the predominance of a particular cell subtype may assist in development of a differential diagnosis.[1]

NONMALIGNANT CONDITIONS
Reactive Neutrophilia

Reactive leukocytosis, an increased WBC count in response to a stress, usually provokes WBC counts between 12,000 and 30,000 cells/mm^3 with a neutrophilic predominance. Catecholamine-induced demargination of neutrophils may result from exercise, surgery, trauma, and even emotional stress. Reid and colleagues[2] evaluated 155 runners postmarathon and found that 100% of them developed a leukocytosis with neutrophilic predominance, likely secondary to demargination of mature neutrophils from the endothelium. Another study, by Nieman and colleagues,[3] reported that leukocyte counts reverted to normal by 24 hours postrace. The same phenomenon can be found in patients who are postictal and postoperative. Reactive leukocytosis is a normal physiologic response but, if leukocytosis persists for greater than 48 hours following a given stressor, further evaluation is recommended.

Acute Infection

Acute infection remains the most common nonmalignant cause of leukocytosis. The acute inflammatory response leads to dilation of small blood vessels, increased vascular permeability, and emigration of leukocytes from circulation to the site of injury.[4] Although circulating neutrophils are the initial responders to acute infection, Furze and Rankin[5] discovered that the bone marrow release of mature granulocytes

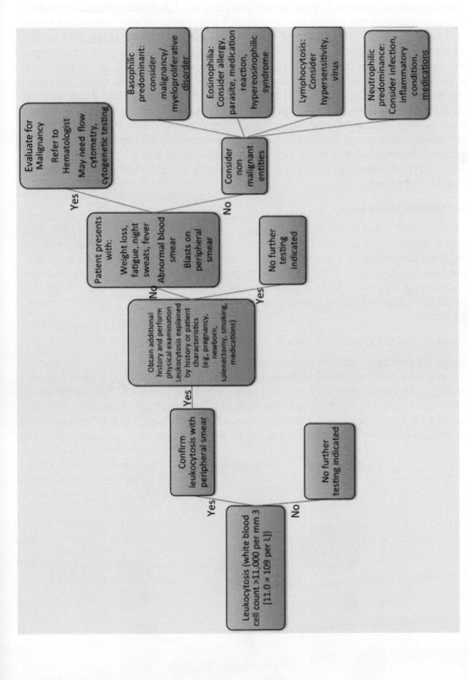

Fig. 1. Evaluation of peripheral leukocytosis.

from storage pools escalates within the first 2 hours following acute insult. In moderate to severe infections, the ongoing stimuli from inflammatory mediators (predominantly interleukin-1 and tumor necrosis factor) enhance both differentiation and proliferation of granulocytic progenitors in the marrow, resulting in a sustained increase in neutrophil production over the course of a few days.[6] The release of immature band forms (**Fig. 2**) and precursor metamyelocytes from the marrow results in a left shift, which may assist in differentiating infection from other nonpathogenic causes of leukocytosis. The presence of toxic granulations and Döhle bodies (**Fig. 3**), small dark blue staining granules and larger gray-blue cytoplasmic inclusions respectively, also suggests that neutrophils are present in response to a bacterial infection.[7] Acute viral infections may also present with short-lived leukocytosis, although it does not often persist as seen in bacterial processes. Any patient presenting with fever and leukocytosis should undergo routine evaluation for common bacterial and viral causes of infection, with work-up to include blood cultures, imaging studies of affected areas, as well as specific viral and bacterial studies that may be consistent with the patient's presenting symptoms.

Bone Marrow Stimulation

Conditions that result in appropriate, physiologic bone marrow stimulation can also cause a leukocytosis. Leukocytosis is frequently seen in the setting of massive blood loss, likely secondary to a combination of inflammation as a result of bleeding, and bone marrow stimulation with increased production of all cell lines.[8] Bone marrow upregulation may also be seen in patients with hemolytic anemia and immune thrombocytopenic purpura, who have chronic red blood cell and platelet losses, respectively.

Inflammation-Mediated Leukocytosis

Chronic inflammation may also result from excessive or unwarranted activation of the immune system from noninfectious causes, including autoimmune disorders, inflammatory bowel disease, and chronic allergic conditions. In many autoimmune diseases, such as rheumatoid arthritis, lupus, and multiple sclerosis, chronic inflammation and resultant leukocytosis are a result of inappropriate activation of the immune response against normal body tissue. Acute and chronic vasculitis

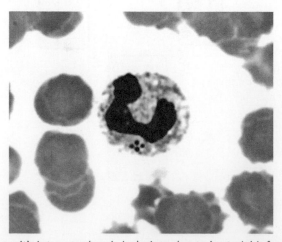

Fig. 2. Band forms with intracytoplasmic inclusions due to bacterial infection.

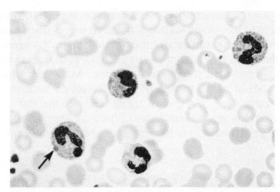

Fig. 3. Toxic granulation and Dohle bodies (*arrow*), suggesting neutrophil response to bacterial infection.

from infectious or autoimmune causes may also cause significant leukocytosis, or disproportionate increase of a particular cell line, as in the case of the absolute eosinophilia seen in Churg-Strauss disease. Although the pathophysiology of inflammatory bowel disease is incompletely understood, part of the chronic inflammation in this condition is attributed to unregulated immune responses against colonizing microbes.[9] Allergic diseases (eg, asthma and chronic urticaria) may also contribute to chronic inflammation through inappropriate immune responses to nonpathogenic external stimuli.[10]

Smoking-Induced Leukocytosis

Cigarette smoking is one of the most common causes of mild leukocytosis and chronic inflammation. Absolute leukocyte count increases in direct proportion to the number of cigarettes smoked daily, as well as in proportion to the total overall number of pack-years, irrespective of cardiovascular risk, respiratory dysfunction, and underlying malignancy. A study of 16,254 men and women 20 to 70 years of age who participated in the Dutch European Prospective Investigation into Cancer and Nutrition (EPIC) subcohort revealed that WBC values were significantly lower with only 24 hours cigarette free before testing, suggesting that smoking-related leukocytosis is likely caused by repeated exposures to an acute stimulus. Notably, that same study discovered that although total WBC count normalized within 2 years of quitting, lymphocytosis and monocytosis often did not resolve until 5 years following smoking cessation.[11] Another study, performed by Abel and colleagues,[12] investigated the hematologic parameters of greater than 461 participants with chemically confirmed smoking cessation and found a sustained decrease in WBC, which they proposed was the result of a decrease in the underlying tobacco-induced inflammation.

Neutrophilia Associated with Asplenia

Asplenic patients frequently show chronic leukocytosis with a neutrophilic predominance. The spleen has a role in the production, distribution, and use of neutrophils. More than 30 years ago, Spencer and colleagues[13] reported that a patient with congenital asplenia had a chronically increased pool of circulating neutrophils as well as increased granulocyte production by the bone marrow. Similar findings were later described in patients who underwent surgical splenectomy. In a study of 96 patients who required splenectomy after traumatic event, 100% of the patients showed postsurgical leukocytosis lasting 5 days, at which point persistent leukocytosis was found only in those with superimposed infections.[14] A separate study found no significant difference in WBC counts even 2 weeks after surgery between patients who developed infection and those who did not. As a consequence, the study suggested using platelet levels in lieu of WBC levels to evaluate for infection in postsplenectomy patients.[15] Beyond surgical and congenital causes, there is growing evidence that the autosplenectomy caused by chronic, silent splenic microinfarctions in sickle cell disease may also cause a chronic, neutrophilic-predominant, leukocytosis.[16]

Medication-Induced Leukocytosis

Several medications have been implicated as causes of benign leukocytosis (**Table 2**). Granulocytes, specifically neutrophils and eosinophils, are the commonly affected cell line. Glucocorticoids are the most common medication-induced cause of leukocytosis, and they provoke an increase in the release of mature neutrophils from bone marrow, as well as decreased adhesion to the endothelial wall, resulting in neutrophil demargination. The increase in WBC count after glucocorticoid administration can occur as quickly as 6 hours after administration, but rarely achieves a level greater than 20,000 cells/μL. Glucocorticoids generally do not result in an increase in less mature (eg, band) forms, so when these cells are present in conjunction with steroid therapy, acute infection should be considered.[17] Exogenously administered epinephrine can also cause demargination of neutrophils and an associated leukocytosis in conjunction with stress response. Lithium has also been found to cause a notable neutrophilia in the setting of chronic use, and was once used as a therapy for chronic neutropenia. At present, granulocyte colony-stimulating factor (G-CSF) agents are used after chemotherapy to shorten the duration of neutropenia, but they often induce an exaggerated bone marrow response, leading to a neutrophilic leukocytosis with or without a left shift.[18]

Acute febrile neutrophilic dermatosis (Sweet syndrome), which presents with skin lesions and fever, may also cause a systemic neutrophilia. Sweet syndrome is strongly associated with acute myelogenous leukemia (AML) and myelodysplastic syndrome (MDS); thus all patients presenting with Sweet syndrome should be evaluated for underlying malignancy. This condition has been linked to several medications, most frequently colony-stimulating factors but also antineoplastic agents, antibiotics, and

Table 2
Medications that may cause leukocytosis

Laboratory Finding	Medications
Neutrophilia	Glucocorticoids, lithium, epinephrine
Sweet syndrome (acute febrile neutrophilic dermatosis)	Colony-stimulating factors, antineoplastic agents, antibiotics, furosemide, antiepileptic agents, oral contraceptives, NSAIDs
Eosinophilia (DRESS Syndrome)	Allopurinol, antiepileptic agents (carbamazepine, phenytoin, lamotrigine), sulfa drugs, antibiotics (minocycline, vancomycin, dapsone)

Abbreviations: DRESS, drug rash with eosinophilia and systemic symptoms; NSAIDs, nonsteroidal antiinflammatory drugs.

contraceptive medications. Drug-induced Sweet syndrome generally resolves with cessation of administration of the offending agent.[19]

Drug rash with eosinophilia and systemic symptoms (DRESS) is another medication-associated syndrome that causes leukocytosis. DRESS is characterized by a morbilliform rash, which may progress to an exfoliative dermatitis, peripheral eosinophilia, and visceral involvement of the lungs, liver, kidneys, or heart. The most common causative agents are antibiotics, anticonvulsants, allopurinol, and sulfa drugs. Treatment involves withdrawal of the offending agent and a prolonged course of glucocorticoids.[20]

Eosinophilia

Eosinophilia is defined as an increased eosinophil count in the peripheral blood (≥500/μL), but there can be wide variations in the degree of increase. Increase in eosinophil count greater than or equal to 20,000/μL is highly concerning for a myelo-proliferative syndrome such as hypereosinophilic syndrome; this requires an immediate evaluation because of pulmonary complications (Löffler syndrome) or cardiac complications (Löffler endocarditis). More mild eosinophilia can be related to allergy syndromes, parasitic infections (discussed later), pulmonary syndromes (asthma), or autoimmune diseases (Churg-Strauss disease).

Helminthic infections

Helminths are complex organisms that remain common causes of chronic and recurrent infections worldwide. Helminth infections (eg, trichinosis, ascariasis, filariasis, and paragonimiasis, strongyloidiasis, toxocariasis) induce immunoglobulin E–mediated immune responses associated with tissue and peripheral eosinophilia, as well as mast cell activation.[21] Complete blood count patterns seen in helminth infections may resemble those found in allergic reactions. Evaluation for this type of organism may be warranted if patients are from endemic areas and present with gastrointestinal symptoms, anemia, or respiratory complaints in conjunction with their eosinophilic leukocytosis (**Table 3**).

HEREDITARY AND CONGENITAL CONDITIONS

Several known rare hereditary and congenital conditions are strongly associated with leukocytosis[22]:

- Hereditary neutrophilia: autosomal dominant condition characterized by WBC counts between 20,000 and 100,000 cells/mm^3, splenomegaly, increased leukocyte alkaline phosphate scores, and widened skull diploe.[23]

Table 3
Conditions associated with increased levels of certain white blood cell subtypes

Cell Line	Conditions Associated with Increased Level
Neutrophils	Infections, inflammatory conditions, reactive, medication induced, bone marrow stimulation
Eosinophils	Allergic conditions, medication reactions, parasitic infections, malignant conditions, dermatologic conditions
Basophils	Leukemias, myeloproliferative disorders, certain allergic conditions
Monocytes	Postsplenectomy, autoimmune disease, viral infections (Epstein-Barr virus in particular), tuberculosis
Lymphocytes	Infections (viral), acute and chronic leukemias

- Familial myeloproliferative disease: syndrome of growth retardation, hepatosplenomegaly, anemia, and leukocytosis, usually leading to childhood death.[24]
- Muckle-Wells syndrome: disease involving flares of skin rash, periodic fever, joint pain, as well as progressive ear and kidney damage.
- Leukocyte adhesion deficiency: patients show persistent leukocytosis (5–20 times normal levels without associated bands), have a history of delayed separation of the umbilical cord, and a stimulus-dependent activation defect of neutrophils leading to recurrent infections.

Children with Down syndrome (trisomy 21) have been found to have transient episodes of leukocytosis that seem to be consistent with acute or chronic leukemia. These children also show recurrent leukemoid reactions with stress and acute illness. Similar findings have also been reported in children who did not have phenotypic characteristics consistent with Down syndrome but were subsequently found to have trisomy 21 mosaicism in the myeloid lineage specifically. However, the underlying cellular mechanism for these leukemoid reactions has not yet been fully characterized.[25]

MALIGNANT CONDITIONS
Hematologic Malignancies

Introduction to clonality
Leukemias and myeloproliferative neoplasms are a result of a clonal proliferation of hematopoietic stem cells within the bone marrow. Nearly all cancers originate from a single cell; this clonal origin is a critical discriminating feature between neoplasia and hyperplasia. There is a subset of diseases in which only a single mutation or translocation is responsible for the development of a malignant clone, such as the BCR-ABL translocation of Chronic Myelogenous Leukemia (CML) or the PML-RARα translocation in acute promyelocytic leukemia . Based on observations of increasing cancer frequency with age, as well as molecular genetic studies, it is thought that a minimum of 5 to 10 accumulated mutations may be necessary for certain malignancies to develop from a normal to a fully malignant phenotype.[26]

Myeloproliferative Disorders

Polycythemia vera (PV), essential thrombocytosis (ET), primary myelofibrosis (PMF), and CML are the 4 recognized myeloproliferative neoplasms. These disorders represent stem cell–derived clonal proliferation. PV, ET, and PMF may all result in leukocytosis, even though the myeloid lineage is not the cell line that is primarily increased in any of these conditions. Because all of these conditions are thought to be associated with genetic mutations with effects early in cell differentiation pathways (eg, JAK-2 and CAL-R), they are not wholly selective of a single lineage.[27] However, in these cases the WBC increase is always seen in conjunction with an increase in another cell line. These diseases also often present with an increased basophil count. With respect to PMF, leukocytosis is generally only seen early in the disease, because all peripheral cell lines decrease as the normal bone marrow is replaced with fibrosis. The most serious complication of all of these conditions is that they have a propensity to transform into AML over time.

Chronic Myelogenous Leukemia

CML is a myeloproliferative disorder arising from clonal proliferation of hematopoietic stem cells. The disease can present in the milder chronic phase or the more concerning acute phase or blast crisis. Most patients present in the chronic phase of the disease and many are asymptomatic. Those who do present with symptoms may have the following complaints:

- Fatigue
- Weight loss
- Bone pain
- Night sweats
- Early satiety (secondary to splenomegaly)

Laboratory evaluation of patients with CML is notable for thrombocytosis, anemia, and a leukocytosis that is often more than 100,000/μL with a prominent left shift. In addition, they have been found to have hyperuricemia, increased serum B_{12} levels, and increased lactate dehydrogenase levels. CML is the first malignancy in which a consistent chromosomal abnormality was discovered. It is a balanced translocation between chromosomes 9 and 22 that creates the Philadelphia chromosome, creating the fusion protein Bcr-Abl. This protein codes for a constitutively active cytoplasmic tyrosine kinase that is thought to be responsible for the chronic phase of the disease. Several tyrosine kinase inhibitors, such as the first-in-class imatinib (Gleevec), target the fusion protein directly and have led to a dramatic improvement in the survival of patients with CML.[28] Most patients who are diagnosed with CML are placed on tyrosine kinase inhibitor therapy as first-line treatment. Curative treatment requires hematopoietic stem cell transplant, which is usually reserved for younger patients who fail tyrosine kinase inhibitors.[29]

Leukemias

Although leukemias are generally managed by hematologist-oncologists, they are often initially detected by primary care physicians. The 4 broad subtypes of leukemia that are most commonly seen are AML, acute lymphoblastic leukemia (ALL), CML (discussed earlier), and chronic lymphocytic leukemia (CLL). These conditions differ in both laboratory studies and clinical presentation, although they are usually readily identified on a peripheral blood smear. All patients suspected of having any leukemic condition should be referred immediately to a hematologist-oncologist for evaluation.

Acute Leukemia

Acute leukemia can be broken down into 2 subtypes: AML and ALL. ALL is predominantly found in children, whereas 80% of adults with acute leukemia have AML. Common symptoms/signs of acute leukemia include:

- Fever
- Night sweats
- Bleeding/bruising
- Fatigue
- Hepatomegaly/splenomegaly (ALL)

Acute leukemia should be suspected when any blasts are seen on the peripheral smear. Diagnosis is formally made with bone marrow biopsy showing greater than 20% blasts. Of note, the patient is not required to have a leukocytosis for the diagnosis of leukemia (**Table 4** provides further information regarding laboratory work-up of leukemia). Treatment of AML in young, fit patients usually involves inpatient chemotherapy for multiple cycles, whereas ALL uses multiple chemotherapy regimens, which can either be given on an inpatient or outpatient basis and entails a total of 2 years of chemotherapy. In otherwise healthy patients with acute leukemia (AML or ALL) and poor prognosis, the standard of care is hematopoietic stem cell transplant.[30]

Table 4
Laboratory evaluation of leukemia

Laboratory Test	Description of Evaluation	Clinical Uses
Peripheral smear	Direct visualization of whole blood under microscope	Identification of blasts in AML and ALL
Bone marrow aspirate/biopsy	Closer examination of hematopoietic stem cells	Evaluate for presence of blasts in acute leukemia, extent of marrow infiltration can aid with prognostication
Cytogenetic testing	Examination of chromosomes via karyotyping and/or FISH	Presence of Philadelphia chromosome in CML or to identify subtypes and prognostic chromosomal mutations in other leukemias
Flow cytometry/ immunophenotyping	Sorting and counting cell populations with specific surface markers	Counting clonal cells to diagnose CLL, diagnose subtypes of acute leukemia
Molecular testing	Testing for mutations at the DNA level by PCR	May identify presence of Philadelphia chromosome in CML, may also identify subtypes of acute leukemia

Abbreviations: FISH, fluorescence in situ hybridization; PCR, polymerase chain reaction.

Chronic Leukemia

CML and CLL are found almost exclusively in adult patients (only 30% of patients with CLL were diagnosed before age 65 years, and <2% of patients before 45 years of age).[31] Compared with acute leukemias, they are indolent and have fewer symptoms.

Chronic Lymphocytic Leukemia

Most patients with CLL are asymptomatic at the time of diagnosis. The diagnosis is most often made when checking routine blood work or for other reasons; however, if made in later stages of disease, patients may present with:

- Weight loss
- Early satiety (secondary to splenomegaly)
- Fatigue
- Petechiae (if thrombocytopenic)
- Recurrent infections (caused by immunodeficiency associated with CLL)

In general, CLL is a very indolent disease. It can often be monitored for a long period of time without need for intervention The diagnosis of CLL requires an absolute clonal B-cell lymphocyte count of greater than 5000/μL.[32] The diagnosis is generally confirmed by flow cytometry, which also provides prognostic markers. As the disease progresses, the development of worsening cytopenias, symptomatic splenomegaly or lymphadenopathy, or markedly increasing WBC counts may require treatment to achieve symptom control. Treatment involves cytotoxic chemotherapy and/or monoclonal antibodies.

Solid Tumors

Some kidney, bladder, lung, and tongue malignancies have been found to secrete G-CSF, thereby causing an increased WBC count with a neutrophilic predominance.

Table 5 Five-year survival by leukemia type		
Type of Malignancy	Age <65 y (%)	Age ≥65 y (%)
AML	44.0	5.8
ALL	72.0	14.7
CML	81.3	37.8
CLL	90.5	76.4

Data from Howlader N, Noone AM, Krapcho M, et al. SEER cancer statistics review, 1975–2013. Bethesda (MD): National Cancer Institute. Available at: http://seer.cancer.gov/csr/1975_2013/. Accessed January 22, 2016, based on November 2015 SEER data submission, posted to the SEER Web site, April 2016.

Solid tumors may also cause leukocytosis when they invade the bone marrow. Tumor invasion of the marrow can result in a leukoerythroblastic reaction, which is characterized by a left-shifted leukocytosis, nucleated red blood cells and other abnormal red cell morphologies, and thrombocytosis seen on peripheral blood smear.[33]

Prognosis and Monitoring Posttreatment

Prognosis for leukemia varies greatly by type of leukemia, age of patient, other comorbid conditions, as well as by cytogenetic characteristics of the leukemia. Survival by type of leukemia is shown in **Table 5**.

Even when leukemia is fully treated and the patient has achieved a complete remission, survivors of leukemia are at risk for several long-term sequelae:

- Second malignancies as a consequence of chemotherapy exposure (particularly with alkylators, anthracyclines, and topoisomerase inhibitors)
- Survivors of ALL may develop osteonecrosis of the large bones
- Decreased cardiac function in patients who received anthracycline therapy
- Metabolic syndrome
- Thyroid function abnormalities
- Gonadal failure

Survivors of acute leukemia as well as those who received hematopoietic stem cell transplant need complete blood count (CBC), electrolyte studies, and endocrine evaluation (hemoglobin A1c, thyroid function testing) at least yearly. Physicians should have a low threshold for echocardiograms, pulmonary function tests, and bone density testing in patients who are symptomatic. Patients with chronic leukemia require CBC monitoring whether they are being treated or monitored. They also require regular physical examinations to evaluate for splenomegaly and lymphadenopathy. Regardless of cancer type, all patients should be kept up to date on vaccinations.[34]

Importantly, patients who have previously been treated for a prior malignancy need to be monitored by standard health care screening practices. Because the goals of therapy are often cure or long-term progression-free survival, patients need to maintain their standard schedules for colonoscopy, mammography, prostate examinations, lung cancer screening, and skin evaluations. These studies are often not ordered or performed by the primary hematologist, and therefore the burden frequently devolves to the primary care physician.

SUMMARY

Leukocytosis is a nonspecific laboratory finding that may be the result of several malignant or nonmalignant causes. Evaluating the patient's medical history, medication regimen, symptom constellation, as well as further laboratory evaluation, including WBC differential, assists in differentiation of the cause of this finding. Commonly, patients with infection; inflammatory conditions, including cigarette smoking; or allergic syndromes may present with a benign leukocytosis. When malignant conditions are suspected, a referral to a hematologist-oncologist should be made for further evaluation.

REFERENCES

1. Munker RHE, Glass J, Paquette R. Modern hematology: biology and clinical management. 2nd edition. New York: Humana Press; 2007.
2. Reid SA, Speedy DB, Thompson JM, et al. Study of hematological and biochemical parameters in runners completing a standard marathon. Clin J Sport Med 2004;14(6):344–53.
3. Nieman DC, Berk LS, Simpson-Westerberg M, et al. Effects of long-endurance running on immune system parameters and lymphocyte function in experienced marathoners. Int J Sports Med 1989;10(5):317–23.
4. Klatt E, Kumar V. Robbins and Cotran review of pathology. 4th edition. New York: Elsevier/Saunders; 2015.
5. Furze RC, Rankin SM. Neutrophil mobilization and clearance in the bone marrow. Immunology 2008;125(3):281–8.
6. Colotta F, Re F, Polentarutti N, et al. Modulation of granulocyte survival and programmed cell death by cytokines and bacterial products. Blood 1992;80(8): 2012–20.
7. Lynch EC. Peripheral blood smear. In: Walker HK, Hall WD, Hurst JW, editors. Clinical methods: The history, physical, and laboratory examinations. 3rd edition. Boston: Butterworths; 1990. p. 732–5.
8. Chalasani N, Patel K, Clark WS, et al. The prevalence and significance of leukocytosis in upper gastrointestinal bleeding. Am J Med Sci 1998;315(4):233–6.
9. Braegger CP, MacDonald TT. Immune mechanisms in chronic inflammatory bowel disease. Ann Allergy 1994;72(2):135–41.
10. Ravin KA, Loy M. The eosinophil in infection. Clin Rev Allergy Immunol 2016; 50(2):214–27.
11. Van Tiel E, Peeters PH, Smit HA, et al. Quitting smoking may restore hematological characteristics within five years. Ann Epidemiol 2002;12(6):378–88.
12. Abel GA, Hays JT, Decker PA, et al. Effects of biochemically confirmed smoking cessation on white blood cell count. Mayo Clin Proc 2005;80(8):1022–8.
13. Spencer RP, McPhedran P, Finch SC, et al. Persistent neutrophilic leukocytosis associated with idiopathic functional asplenia. J Nucl Med 1972;13(3):224–6.
14. Weng J, Brown CV, Rhee P, et al. White blood cell and platelet counts can be used to differentiate between infection and the normal response after splenectomy for trauma: prospective validation. J Trauma 2005;59(5):1076–80.
15. Banerjee A, Kelly KB, Zhou HY, et al. Diagnosis of infection after splenectomy for trauma should be based on lack of platelets rather than white blood cell count. Surg Infect (Larchmt) 2014;15(3):221–6.
16. Brousse V, Buffet P, Rees D. The spleen and sickle cell disease: the sick(led) spleen. Br J Haematol 2014;166(2):165–76.
17. Dale DC, Fauci AS, Guerry DI, et al. Comparison of agents producing a neutrophilic leukocytosis in man. hydrocortisone, prednisone, endotoxin, and etiocholanolone. J Clin Invest 1975;56(4):808–13.

18. Mintzer DM, Billet SN, Chmielewski L. Drug-induced hematologic syndromes. Adv Hematol 2009;2009:495863.
19. Cohen PR. Sweet's syndrome–a comprehensive review of an acute febrile neutrophilic dermatosis. Orphanet J Rare Dis 2007;2:34.
20. Tas S, Simonart T. Management of drug rash with eosinophilia and systemic symptoms (DRESS syndrome): an update. Dermatology 2003;206(4):353–6.
21. Shin MH, Lee YA, Min DY. Eosinophil-mediated tissue inflammatory responses in helminth infection. Korean J Parasitol 2009;47(Suppl):S125–31.
22. Berliner N. Leukocytosis and leukopenia. In: Goldman L, Schafer A, editors. Goldman-Cecil medicine. 25th edition. New York: Elsevier/Saunders; 2016. p. 1129–38.
23. Herring WB, Smith LG, Walker RI, et al. Hereditary neutrophilia. Am J Med 1974; 56(5):729–34.
24. Randall DL, Reiquam CW, Githens JH, et al. Familial myeloproliferative disease. a new syndrome closely simulating myelogenous leukemia in childhood. Am J Dis Child 1965;110(5):479–500.
25. Weinstein HJ. Congenital leukaemia and the neonatal myeloproliferative disorders associated with Down's syndrome. Clin Haematol 1978;7(1):147–54.
26. Kasper DFA, Hauser S, Longo D, et al. Harrison's principles of internal medicine. 19th edition. New York: McGraw-Hill Education/Medical; 2015.
27. Levine RL, Gilliland DG. Myeloproliferative disorders. Blood 2008;112(6):2190–8.
28. Bansal A, Radich J. Is cure for chronic myeloid leukemia possible in the tyrosine kinase inhibitors era? Curr Opin Hematol 2016;23(2):115–20.
29. Moen MD, McKeage K, Plosker GL, et al. Imatinib: a review of its use in chronic myeloid leukaemia. Drugs 2007;67(2):299–320.
30. Hoffman RBE, Silberstein LE, Heslop HE, et al. Hematology: basic principles and practice. 6th edition. Philadelphia: Saunders/Elsevier; 2013.
31. Howlader N, Noone AM, Krapcho M, et al. SEER cancer statistics review, 1975-2012. Bethesda (MD): National Cancer Institute; based on November 2014 SEER data submission, posted to the SEER Web site, April 2015.
32. Lin T, Awan F, Byrd J. Chronic lymphocytic leukemia. In: Hoffman R, Benz EJ, Silberstein LE, et al, editors. Hematology: basic principles and practice. 6th edition. Elsevier; 2013. p. 1170–91.
33. George TI. Malignant or benign leukocytosis. Hematology Am Soc Hematol Educ Program 2012;2012:475–84.
34. Davis AS, Viera AJ, Mead MD. Leukemia: an overview for primary care. Am Fam Physician 2014;89(9):731–8.

Polycythemia and Thrombocytosis

Aric Parnes, MD[a,b],*, Arvind Ravi, MD, PhD[b]

KEYWORDS

- Myeloproliferative neoplasms • Polycythemia vera • Essential thrombocytosis
- Myelofibrosis • *JAK2* mutation

KEY POINTS

- Polycythemia vera (PV) involves excess red blood cell production, whereas essential thrombocytosis (ET) involves an excess of platelets.
- The myeloproliferative neoplasms (MPNs) share underlying mutations, particularly *JAK2V617F*, seen in nearly all cases of PV and roughly half of all cases of ET and myelofibrosis.
- Although some patients present with generalized symptoms and splenomegaly, many are asymptomatic at presentation and are identified by routine laboratory testing.
- The mainstay of PV therapy is phlebotomy and low-dose aspirin, although for both PV and ET cytoreductive agents and selective JAK2 inhibitors (ruxolitinib) may also be used.
- Patients with PV and ET are at risk for both thrombotic and hemorrhagic complications, and a subset of patients progress to myelofibrosis and acute myeloid leukemia, leading to a worsened prognosis.

INTRODUCTION

Overview

Myeloproliferative neoplasms (MPNs) are a group of disorders marked by abnormal proliferation of immature and mature myeloid cells from the bone marrow. They are driven by the presence of an abnormal neoplastic stem cell clone that gives rise to excess red blood cells (RBCs), white blood cells, and/or platelets. This clone is presumed to harbor underlying genetic mutations that confer unchecked growth and proliferation.[1]

Classification

In the past, MPNs have been separated into those diseases involving the *BCR-ABL1* gene fusion (also known as the Philadelphia chromosome, a marker of chronic

Disclosure: The authors have nothing to disclose.
[a] Division of Hematology, Brigham and Women's Hospital, 75 Francis Street, Boston, MA 02115, USA; [b] Dana-Farber Cancer Institute, 450 Brookline Avenue, Boston, MA 02215, USA
* Corresponding author. Brigham and Women's Hospital, 75 Francis Street, Boston, MA 02115.
E-mail address: aparnes@partners.org

Prim Care Clin Office Pract 43 (2016) 589–605
http://dx.doi.org/10.1016/j.pop.2016.07.011
0095-4543/16/© 2016 Elsevier Inc. All rights reserved.
primarycare.theclinics.com

myelogenous leukemia [CML]; See Page Widick and Eric S. Winer's article, "Leukocytosis and Leukemia", in this issue) from those that do not, such as polycythemia vera (PV), essential thrombocytosis (ET), and myelofibrosis (MF).

Although PV is defined by increased erythrocyte level and ET is defined by increased platelet level, there can be a degree of clinical overlap (**Table 1**).[1]

Genetics

The clinical resemblance of MPNs has led to a long-standing suspicion that these disorders have a shared genetic basis. Since the advent of gene sequencing, several genetic mutations have been identified in both PV and ET, improving the understanding of the molecular biology of these diseases.

The most common mutation in these cases targets the protein Janus kinase 2 (JAK2), a nonreceptor tyrosine kinase. JAK2 helps mediate signals from outside the cell to drive growth and differentiation. When cytokine receptors bind to ligands (erythropoietin [Epo], thrombopoietin, or interleukins) they induce phosphorylation of JAK2, which then activates downstream signaling cascades to cause transcription of new genes (**Fig. 1**).[2]

The most frequently seen mutation is *JAK2V617F* (in exon 14), which inactivates an inhibitory domain of the protein to trigger cytokine independent growth. This mutation is seen in nearly all cases of PV, as well as more than half of all ET and MF cases (**Fig. 2**). The remaining 4% of PV cases without this classic mutation typically harbor alternative mutations in JAK2 exon 12.[2,3]

The burden of JAK2 mutations in ET and primary myelofibrosis is less than for PV, estimated at 50% to 60%, with an additional 25% attributed to calreticulin (CALR) mutations, and 5% attributed to myeloproliferative leukemia protein (MPL) mutations. The remaining 15% are termed triple negative.[1,4–6] These 3 mutations are mutually exclusive.

POLYCYTHEMIA VERA
Definition

PV is a clonal disorder of excess RBC production by the bone marrow.

Epidemiology

- Between 1 and 40 per 100,000 people
- Slight male predominance
- Median age of mid-60s at diagnosis
- Familial pattern in only rare cases[1,4,7]

Table 1
Classification of MPNs

Myeloproliferative Neoplasm (MPN)	Hallmark
Philadelphia Chromosome (*BCR-ABL1*) Positive	
CML	Excess white blood cells
Philadelphia Chromosome (BCR-ABL1) Negative	
PV	Excess RBCs
ET	Excess platelets
MF	Megakaryocyte proliferation within a fibrotic bone marrow

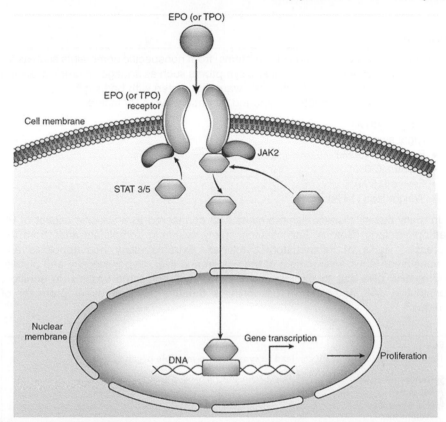

Fig. 1. Many of the mutations in PV and ET relate to growth factor signaling in myeloid cells. Signals from outside the cell (eg, Epo, thrombopoietin), bind to growth factor receptors, which together with JAK2 activate a series of downstream pathways. The JAK2V617F mutation leads to constitutive signaling, driving growth and proliferation of mutant cells. EPO, erythropoietin; STAT, signal transducer and activator of transcription; TPO, thrombopoetin. (*Adapted from* Saeidi K. Myeloproliferative neoplasms: current molecular biology and genetics. Crit Rev Oncol Hematol 2016;98:375–89.)

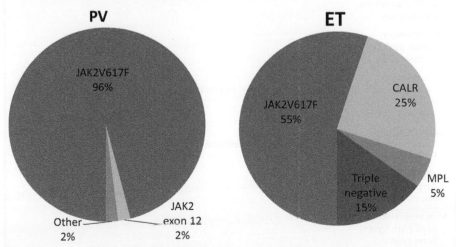

Fig. 2. JAK2 mutations are found in almost all PV cases as well as roughly half of all cases of ET.

Presentation

Patients with PV report a range of symptoms, from nonspecific complaints such as fatigue and night sweats, to more classic symptoms such as aquagenic pruritus, an itch triggered by water contact (particularly warm/hot water) with bathing.[8]

Common systemic symptoms reported by patients with PV include:

- Fatigue (80%)
- Night sweats (50%)
- Bone pain (50%)
- Pruritus (50%)
- Fevers (15%)
- Weight loss (13%)

In many cases, disease symptoms can be connected to a specific aspect of PV pathophysiology (**Box 1**). For instance, many systemic complaints arise from the increased levels of inflammatory cytokines. Extramedullary hematopoiesis and sequestration drive enlargement of the spleen and liver. Hyperviscosity and platelet aggregation give rise to thromboses in both small and large vessels. In addition, constitutive JAK activation in basophils is thought to be a direct promoter of pruritus.[9–12]

Box 1
The pathophysiology of PV can lead to symptoms in multiple organ systems

Systemic
  Fatigue
  Night sweats
  Weight loss
  Fevers

Neurologic
  Headaches
  Visual disturbance
  Tinnitus
  Difficulty concentrating
  Dizziness
  Lightheadedness
  Paresthesias

Genitourinary
  Sexual dysfunction
  Nephrolithiasis (uric acid stones)

Dermatologic
  Erythromelalgia (erythema plus burning in extremities, particularly the palms and soles)
  Pruritus
  Raynaud

Gastrointestinal
  Abdominal discomfort (organomegaly/thrombosis)
  Early satiety

Cardiovascular
  Atypical chest pain
  Palpitations

Musculoskeletal
  Joint pain (gout)
  Bone pain

Not featured in this list of symptoms is thromboembolic disease, including stroke, myocardial infarction, deep vein thrombosis, and pulmonary embolism. Although these are often misconstrued as late manifestations, patients commonly present with these complications. These complications result in symptoms including focal neurologic deficits, chest pain, dyspnea, syncope, and limb pain or swelling.

Another common presentation is the finding of increased RBC count found on routine laboratory work in an asymptomatic patient.

Differential Diagnosis

Several elements in the history and physical examination can alert clinicians to consider PV:

- Increased RBC count
- Hepatomegaly/splenomegaly
- Aquagenic pruritus
- Abdominal thrombosis (portal/splenic/hepatic vein)
- Plethora/ruddy complexion

Because half of all cases of erythrocytosis are secondary, careful attention must be paid to exclude common alternative causes of increased RBC count, such as sleep apnea, lung disease, and smoking (**Box 2**).[13]

Diagnostic Approach

The official 2008 World Health Organization (WHO) diagnosis of PV involves a combination of criteria including:[14]

- Increased hemoglobin level
- JAK2 mutation status
- Low Epo level
- Hypercellular bone marrow (**Box 3**)

For patients with persistent erythrocytosis and who do not have an obvious secondary cause, the authors suggest an initial test for the *JAK2V617F* mutation as well as an Epo level (**Fig. 3**). If mutation testing is negative but Epo level is low or clinical

---

Box 2
Erythrocytosis can be caused by several different conditions

Polycythemia vera (or other MPN)

Sleep apnea/obesity hypoventilation

Structural heart disease

Chronic lung disease

Renal artery stenosis

Medications (diuretics, androgens, TKIs)

Exogenous drugs (Epo)

Neoplasms (renal, hepatocellular carcinoma)

Smoking

Rarely familial/congenital (hemoglobin mutations)

Abbreviation: TKIs, tyrosine kinase inhibitors.

> **Box 3**
> **Revised 2008 WHO criteria for PV, involving a combination of serum testing, mutation analysis, and bone marrow pathology. Diagnosis requires both major and 1 minor criterion or the first major and 2 minor criteria**
>
> Major criteria
> 1. Increased RBC volume (typically hemoglobin level >18.5 g/dL in men or >16.5 g/dL in women)
> 2. Presence of *JAK2V617F* or other functionally similar mutation
>
> Minor criteria
> 1. Bone marrow biopsy showing hypercellularity with trilineage growth
> 2. Serum Epo level less than the reference range for normal
> 3. Endogenous erythroid colony formation in vitro
>
> *Adapted from* Tefferi A, Thiele J, Orazi A, et al. Proposals and rationale for revision of the World Health Organization diagnostic criteria for polycythemia vera, essential thrombocythemia, and primary myelofibrosis: recommendations from an ad hoc international expert panel. Blood 2007;110:1093.

suspicion remains high, it is worth additionally testing for the JAK2 exon 12 mutation along with referral to hematology for possible bone marrow biopsy and further management. In contrast, a normal to increased Epo level should trigger reevaluation of congenital or acquired causes of erythrocytosis.[1,5]

Even though bone marrow biopsy remains part of the WHO diagnostic criteria, with the advent of genetic testing for MPNs, bone marrow biopsy is frequently omitted unless primary or secondary myelofibrosis or transformation to leukemia is being considered.

When to Refer

- Low Epo level or confirmed JAK2 mutation suggestive of PV
- Concern for possible complications of PV in a patient with increased RBC count (particularly new thrombotic/hemorrhagic events)
- More urgent triage as warranted by clinical presentation (eg, PE)

Treatment

The central tenet of treatment of PV focuses on reducing the risk of thromboembolic disease. Not all patients require cytoreductive therapy, only high-risk patients, but all patients should be started on either antiplatelet therapy or anticoagulation unless they are bleeding. Typically, low-dose aspirin is adequate unless the patient has already had a thrombotic event.[15,16]

Once the diagnosis of PV is made, a risk assessment must be completed. High-risk patients include those aged greater than 60 years or with a history of thrombosis.[17] Other factors suspected of increasing risk include cardiovascular risk factors (cardiovascular disease, diabetes, hypertension, hyperlipidemia, smoking) and leukocytosis,[18,19] but consensus regarding their importance has not yet been reached.

Low-risk patients do not need cytoreduction, but still warrant low-dose aspirin to prevent blood clots, both arterial and venous. The erythrocytosis can be managed by periodic phlebotomy to maintain a hematocrit less than 45% in men and less than 42% in women.[20] Phlebotomy can be done up to twice a week, with 1 unit of RBCs taken off each time. Side effects that patients may incur, especially if phlebotomy is frequent, include fatigue, dizziness, orthostatic hypotension, and syncope. The essence of phlebotomy is to cause iron deficiency, so blood production slows. Thus,

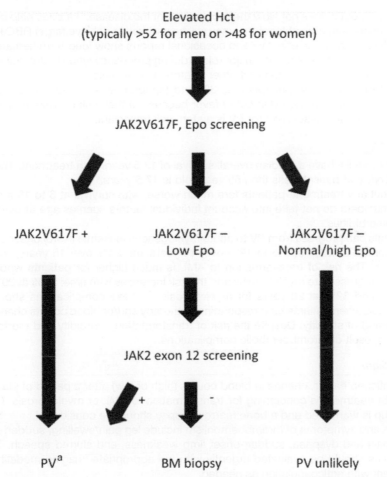

Elevated Hct
(typically >52 for men or >48 for women)

JAK2V617F, Epo screening

JAK2V617F +

JAK2V617F −
Low Epo

JAK2V617F −
Normal/high Epo

JAK2 exon 12 screening

+   −

PV^a   BM biopsy   PV unlikely

Fig. 3. Diagnostic algorithm for the evaluation of PV. When PV is unlikely, alternate causes of erythrocytosis should be re-evaluated. [a]Note that borderline increase in RBC can also be from ET. BM, bone marrow; Hct, hematocrit.

iron replacement should not be given unless anemia ensues and even then it must be done cautiously to avoid the return of polycythemia.

High-risk patients, either aged more than 60 years or having a history of thrombo-embolic disease, as mentioned earlier should be considered for cytoreductive therapy with or without phlebotomy as needed.[17] Other indications for cytoreduction include persistent symptoms despite phlebotomy, poor tolerance of phlebotomy, or platelet count greater than $1.5 \times 10^6/\mu L$. First-line cytoreduction uses hydroxyurea. Downregulating blood production, hydroxyurea's primary side-effect is predictably myelosuppression. Other nonspecific side effects can occur, such as fatigue, headache, and rash. Otherwise it tends to be well tolerated. Slow titration of the dose is essential because hydroxyurea's effect on blood counts is delayed by days, and even weeks.

A new second-line therapy option is ruxolitinib, which was US Food and Drug Administration approved in 2015 for hydroxyurea-intolerant patients or refractory disease. Ruxolitinib is a JAK1/JAK2 inhibitor and works well in reducing symptoms and spleen size, but it does not slow the progression of the disease.[21] It does help control blood counts, although phlebotomy may still be required to achieve target RBC levels.

Interferon alfa is also effective and occasional reports show long-term hematologic and molecular remissions.[22] Its major role is during pregnancy when hydroxyurea and ruxolitinib are contraindicated or if other treatments have failed.

Busulfan, radioactive phosphorous-32, and pipobroman are treatments that are infrequently used, having fallen out of favor because of their risk of leukemogenesis.

The treatment of last resort for PV is a stem cell transplant.

Prognosis

Patients with PV have a median overall survival of 13.5 years with treatment. The median survival of patients less than 65 years old is 17.5 years.[23]

Without any treatment, patients fare much worse, with survival at 6 to 18 months. These numbers do not take into account individual factors such as age at diagnosis and comorbidities.

Patients can progress from PV to acute myelogenous leukemia (AML) or secondary myelofibrosis at rates of 6% to 19% over 15 years and 24% over 15 years, respectively.[23,24] The risk of transformation to AML is much higher for patients who have already progressed to myelofibrosis and the risk increases with time: 24% at 20 years for AML and 32% at 20 years for myelofibrosis.[24] These complications should be considered when patients stop responding to therapy and/or blood counts change after a period of stability. Despite the risk of transformation, morbidity and mortality is mostly a result of thromboembolic complications.

Alarm Signs

As mentioned earlier, change in blood counts (high or low) after a period of stabilization with treatment is concerning for transformation to AML or myelofibrosis. Closer follow-up is warranted and a bone marrow biopsy should be considered.

Signs and symptoms of thromboembolism include leg pain/swelling, sudden-onset chest pain and dyspnea, sudden-onset limb weakness, and slurred speech. These symptoms should be evaluated urgently with the appropriate imaging modality and treatment with anticoagulation as needed.

ESSENTIAL THROMBOCYTOSIS
Definition

ET involves an excess of platelet production by the bone marrow.

Epidemiology

- From 1 to 50 per 100,000 people
- Female predominance
- Median age of 60s at diagnosis
- Familial pattern in only rare cases[1,4]

Presentation

Patients with ET report a variety of symptoms that largely overlap with those of PV, including fatigue, weight loss, and night sweats, and with splenomegaly on examination. Similar to PV, ET also increases the risk of thrombotic events, occurring in 2% to 4% of patients.

ET in particular can also be associated with hemorrhagic complications. Common bleeding complications include:

- Epistaxis
- Gingival bleeding
- Easy bruising

Other sources of bleeding, such as gastrointestinal hemorrhage, are usually rare. However, they can be seen in patients with exceptionally high platelet counts $(1.5 \times 10^6/\mu L)$. In these cases, increased bleeding is likely a result of acquired von Willebrand disease.[12]

Differential Diagnosis

ET is suspected when the platelet count is greater than the upper limit of normal. However, a careful history and physical examination are warranted in the initial evaluation, because thrombocytosis most commonly has secondary causes, such as acute inflammation/infection, splenectomy, or iron deficiency (**Box 4**).[4,5]

Diagnostic Approach

The revised 2008 WHO criteria for ET include a combination of:

- Increased platelet counts
- Clonal genetic markers (eg, *JAK2V617F*)
- Bone marrow biopsy
- Exclusion of other causes (**Box 5**)[14]

If concerned about a platelet count that remains increased in the absence of secondary causes, the authors suggest moving forward with genetic testing. In the past, *JAK2V617F* mutation analysis was typically done first. However, with the recent discovery of the prominent role of CALR in up to one-third of cases and the advent of rapid genetic panel testing through next-generation sequencing, the authors have begun testing with larger gene panels that contain JAK2, CALR, and MPL in order to reduce diagnostic delays and simplify the algorithm. Panel testing for gene sequencing may increase cost. However, it has the ability to enhance diagnostic, prognostic, and eventually therapeutic capabilities. Regardless of the results of mutation testing, if clinical suspicion for ET exists, the authors suggest referral to

---

Box 4
Secondary causes to be considered when evaluating a patient with new thrombocytosis

Differential diagnosis for increased platelet counts

Essential thrombocytosis (or other MPN)

Iron deficiency

Postsplenectomy

Postsurgery

Infections

Inflammatory disorders

Other neoplasms

Hemolysis

Trauma

Congenital mutations (rare)

Box 5
Revised 2008 WHO criteria for ET. All 4 criteria must be met to establish a diagnosis of ET

1. Sustained platelet count greater than or equal to $450 \times 10^9/L$

2. Bone marrow biopsy showing mainly megakaryocyte lineage proliferation

3. Not meeting WHO criteria for other myeloid neoplasms

4. JAK2V617F (or other clonal marker) or no evidence of reactive thrombocytosis

Adapted from Tefferi A, Thiele J, Orazi A, et al. Proposals and rationale for revision of the World Health Organization diagnostic criteria for polycythemia vera, essential thrombocythemia, and primary myelofibrosis: recommendations from an ad hoc international expert panel. Blood 2007;110:1094.

---

hematology for possible bone marrow biopsy because genetic analysis alone cannot distinguish ET from other MPNs (eg, prefibrotic primary myelofibrosis [PMF]). A complete diagnostic algorithm is shown in **Fig. 4.**[3–5]

Even though bone marrow biopsy remains part of the WHO diagnostic criteria and the degree of fibrosis in the marrow can be prognostic, with the advent of genetic testing for MPNs, in practice bone marrow biopsy is frequently omitted unless primary or secondary myelofibrosis or transformation to leukemia is being considered. Importantly, at times only a bone marrow biopsy can differentiate between essential thrombocythemia and myelofibrosis.

When to Refer

- Persistent thrombocytosis in the absence of a clear secondary cause
- Mutation-positive or mutation-negative thrombocytosis concerning for ET

Treatment

Similar to treatment of PV, treatment of essential thrombocythemia is also risk based. Risk factors for thrombosis have been well defined and validated for a scoring system called IPSET (International Prognostic Score for thrombosis in Essential Thrombocythemia).[25–27] This scoring system uses age greater than 60 years (1 point), history of thrombosis (2 points), cardiovascular risk factors (1 point), and JAK2 mutation status (2 points) to reach a total score that correlates with risk of thrombosis. Low risk is defined as less than 2 points in total (1.03% patients per year); intermediate risk, 2 points (2.35% patients per year); and high risk as more than 2 points (3.56% patients per year). Other risk factors are not as well defined and therefore are not included in this scoring system: leukocytosis, presence of symptoms, allele burden, other concurrent mutations, and so forth. Cytoreductive therapy should be started for patients at high risk for thrombosis, with platelet count greater than $1.5 \times 10^6/\mu L$, or with acquired von Willebrand disease or other symptoms.

Previous randomized control trials showed hydroxyurea to be superior to placebo or anagrelide in reducing the risk of thrombosis.[28,29] These trials have led to the use of hydroxyurea as the preferred agent for cytoreduction. Myelosuppression is the most important side effect, so the treatment strategy is the same as for PV: slow titration to avoid overshooting and associated cytopenias.

Anagrelide is a reasonable second-line therapeutic choice, although its efficacy may be diminished in patients with CALR mutation.[30] It works by decreasing megakaryocyte differentiation. Caution is needed in patients with cardiac disease because anagrelide may trigger palpitations, arrhythmias, and edema.

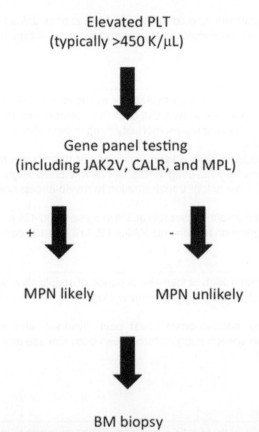

Elevated PLT
(typically >450 K/µL)

Gene panel testing
(including JAK2V, CALR, and MPL)

+   −

MPN likely   MPN unlikely

BM biopsy

Fig. 4. Diagnostic algorithm for the evaluation of ET. Note that even if mutations are found, a bone marrow biopsy may be required to distinguish ET from another MPN, such as PMF.

Interferon also is effective and the newer pegylated interferon has an easier dosing schedule (once a week) and is better tolerated. However, side effects are still common and include fatigue, flulike symptoms (very common), myelosuppression, depression, and autoimmune disease. For patients with a history of mental health disorders, interferon should be avoided. The best role for interferon is still debated because in a subset of patients it can induce long-term remissions and complete molecular responses regardless of the underlying mutation.[31,32] An ongoing clinical trial is comparing interferon with hydroxyurea in order to determine which drug is the preferred first line. In the meantime, standard of care remains hydroxyurea when cytoreduction and risk reduction are necessary.[33] Of note, interferon is the treatment of choice for patients with MPN who are pregnant.

Potential future second-line therapy may eventually include JAK2 inhibitors such as ruxolitinib. Ruxolitinib is not approved for essential thrombocythemia, but reports have shown it to decrease JAK2 allele burden over time, including 2 cases of a complete molecular remission.[34] Drugs used in the past to treat ET, such as busulfan, pipobroman, and P-32, have fallen out of favor because of their leukemogenesis.

The only cure to date is via stem cell transplant, a treatment that is difficult to justify for most patients given their overall good prognosis.

In addition, all patients should take low-dose aspirin unless they have active bleeding. Anticoagulation should be substituted or added if they have a past history of thrombosis.

Prognosis

Despite the risk of transformation to AML or myelofibrosis, life expectancy is near normal,[35] but not completely normal. Out of all the myeloproliferative diseases, essential thrombocythemia has the lowest mortality[23] regardless of mutation, with a median survival of 19.8 years.

CALR-positive patients have a lower incidence of thrombosis than JAK2-positive patients even though they have higher platelet counts on average. MPL-positive patients may have a higher risk of transformation to myelofibrosis compared with other mutations.[23]

Overall the risk of myelofibrosis is low at 3% in 5 years and 4% to 15% in 15 years,[36] as is the risk of progression to leukemia (AML): 1% to 3% in 10 years, 8% in 20 years.[37]

Alarm Signs

Change in blood counts (high or low) after a period of stabilization with treatment suggests progression of disease. A bone marrow biopsy may be the only means of establishing why.

Leg pain/swelling, sudden-onset chest pain, dyspnea, and sudden-onset limb weakness or slurred speech suggest thromboembolic disease and should be investigated urgently.

MYELOFIBROSIS
Definition

Myelofibrosis is defined by fibrotic changes in the bone marrow, which can be associated with ineffective hematopoiesis and marrow failure.

PMF refers to cases of myelofibrosis that cannot be attributed to progression from another process, such as PV or ET.

Overview

Myelofibrosis is a clinically important MPN with similar features to PV and ET. Despite this overlap, MF can be thought of as more advanced on the spectrum of MPNs, representing a state of ineffective hematopoiesis and progressive bone marrow failure. Its prognosis is worse than the other MPNs, in part because of progression to AML (See Page Widick and Eric S. Winer's article, "Leukocytosis and Leukemia", in this issue). At present, bone marrow transplant is the only potentially curative therapy.

Classification

There are 2 broad classes of myelofibrosis:

- Primary myelofibrosis (no clear preceding MPN or other disease)
- Secondary myelofibrosis (progressed from another disease, such as PV or ET)

Global rates of myelofibrosis are roughly comparable with other MPNs, affecting roughly 1 in 100,000 individuals. The mutational spectrum is closest to that of ET, with genetic analyses showing JAK2 (65%), CALR (25%), and MPL (7%) mutations and the rest called triple negative.[5,38]

Presentation

Although symptoms overlap with those of patients with PV and ET, patients with myelofibrosis tend to have more severe constitutional symptoms, such as fatigue and weight loss. They also have greater rates of splenomegaly (90%) and hepatomegaly (70%) caused by extramedullary hematopoiesis.[12] Other specific features that warrant closer investigation include:

- Jaundice, spider angiomas, and encephalopathy, suggesting liver dysfunction
- Localizing back pain, suggesting osteosclerosis or periostitis

Diagnosis

The revised 2008 WHO criteria for PMF involve a combination of laboratory, genetic, and clinical features (**Box 6**).

Unlike the other myeloproliferative diseases, myelofibrosis ultimately requires a bone marrow biopsy for diagnosis because other features of these diseases can be similar and there is no other means of finding fibrosis in the marrow.

The diagnostic criteria for myelofibrosis highlight some of the challenges of myeloproliferative disease. The clinical and laboratory features of PV, ET, and MF overlap, including the genetics. Degrees of marrow fibrosis can be present in each MPN (see **Fig. 5**), as can extramedullary hematopoiesis. However, splenomegaly in myelofibrosis is more common and some clinicians have argued that it should be a major criterion.[39] Early phases of disease may lack some of the classic features and the natural course of each can morph into others. These features make the myeloproliferative diseases fascinating and an promising area of research.

Management

The management for myelofibrosis is more challenging than it is for other myeloproliferative diseases. The reason for this is 2-fold. One is poor responses to treatment and the second is that treatment frequently causes a decrease in blood counts when

---

Box 6
Revised 2008 WHO criteria for diagnosis of PMF. Diagnosis requires meeting all 3 major and 2 minor criteria

Major criteria
1. Presence of megakaryocyte proliferation and atypia with marrow fibrosis, or, in the absence of significant reticulin fibrosis, megakaryocyte changes accompanied by an increased bone marrow cellularity with granulocytic proliferation and often decreased erythropoiesis (**Fig. 5**)
2. Not meeting WHO criteria for alternative MPNs
3. Presence of *JAK2 617VF* or other clonal marker, or no alternative inflammatory/neoplastic cause of fibrosis

Minor criteria
1. Leukoerythroblastosis (myelophthisic smear): teardrop RBCs, immature granulocytes (left shift), and nucleated RBCs (**Fig. 6**)
2. Increased lactate dehydrogenase level
3. Anemia
4. Palpable splenomegaly

Adapted from Tefferi A, Thiele J, Orazi A, et al. Proposals and rationale for revision of the World Health Organization diagnostic criteria for polycythemia vera, essential thrombocythemia, and primary myelofibrosis: recommendations from an ad hoc international expert panel. Blood 2007;110:1095.

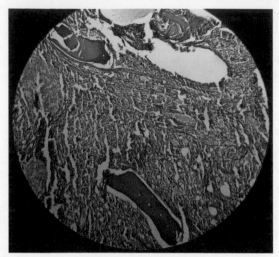

Fig. 5. A bone marrow biopsy stained for reticulin fibrosis (seen as dark brown/black lines). Note that few hematopoietic cells are seen because the marrow has been replaced by fibrosis (reticulin stain, original magnification ×20).

significant cytopenias already exist. For this reason, the use of hydroxyurea is not always helpful. Since ruxolitinib came on the market in 2011, it has become the first-line therapy and is effective in patients with or without a JAK2 mutation.[40,41] However, the benefit is limited to symptom improvement and spleen size reduction. It has also been shown to improve quality of life, but may have little effect on the progression of disease. The 3-year follow-up to the COMFORT-II (Controlled Myelofibrosis Study With Oral Janus-associated Kinase Inhibitor Treatment) study showed a survival improvement.[42,43] Similar to hydroxyurea, patients also frequently have an initial decline in blood counts before any improvement.

Erythropoietin-stimulating agents and androgens such as danazol can be helpful early on to improve anemia. Frequently the mainstay of therapeutic intervention is supportive care with regular RBC and/or platelet transfusions.

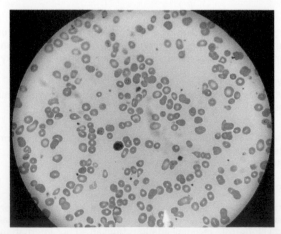

Fig. 6. Leukoerythroblastosis (myelophthisic smear) showing teardrop cells and a nucleated RBC.

Stem cell transplant, reserved for higher-risk disease, remains the only option for a possible cure, but is limited to a few patients because of its risk of complications like graft-versus-host disease, infections, and other transplant-related morbidity. Treatment of primary and secondary types of myelofibrosis is generally the same. Patients should be encouraged to participate in clinical trials to advance the understanding and treatment options available for this difficult disease.

Prognosis

Features associated with a worse prognosis in myelofibrosis include:

- Age greater than 65 years
- Constitutional symptoms
- White blood cell count greater than 25 K/µL
- Circulating blasts greater than 1%
- Platelet count less than 100 K/µL
- Hemoglobin less than 10 g/dL
- Transfusion dependence

The most frequent causes of death in patients are infection, thrombosis, hemorrhage caused by progressive marrow failure, and acute leukemia, which occurs in 10% to 20% of patients.[11] However, such cases of transformation to AML are associated with worse prognosis than de novo AML, and survival is typically in the range of months. Myelofibrosis has a worse overall prognosis (5.9-year median survival)[23] than the other myeloproliferative diseases.

SUMMARY

With the advent of modern molecular biology, the similar clinical pictures of PV and ET have been shown to have a common molecular basis, with shared mutations of growth factor signaling in early myeloid cells. Many of the clinical symptoms that follow are related to a shared pathophysiology of chronic inflammation and prothrombotic state.

Although treatment options are currently limited to cytoreductive therapies and JAK2 inhibitors, several therapies are being developed. In the rare cases in which these disorders progress to more advanced disease states such as myelofibrosis or AML, the gold standard of therapy remains bone marrow transplant.

REFERENCES

1. Aruch D, Mascarenhas J. Contemporary approach to essential thrombocythemia and polycythemia vera. Curr Opin Hematol 2016;23(2):150–60.
2. Anderson LA, McMullin MF. Epidemiology of MPN: what do we know? Curr Hematol Malig Rep 2014;9:340–9.
3. Azzato EM, Bagg A. Molecular genetic evaluation of myeloproliferative neoplasms. Int J Lab Hematol 2015;37(Suppl 1):61–71.
4. Tefferi A, Barbui T. Essential thrombocythemia and polycythemia vera: focus on clinical practice. Mayo Clin Proc 2015;90:1283–93.
5. Tefferi A, Pardanani A. Myeloproliferative neoplasms: a contemporary review. JAMA Oncol 2015;1:97–105.
6. Barosi G. Essential thrombocythemia vs. early/prefibrotic myelofibrosis: why does it matter. Best Pract Res Clin Haematol 2014;27:129–40.
7. Titmarsh GJ, Duncombe AS, McMullin MF, et al. How common are myeloproliferative neoplasms? A systematic review and meta-analysis. Am J Hematol 2014;89:581–7.

8. Weisshaar E, Weiss M, Mettang T, et al. Paraneoplastic itch: an expert position statement from the Special Interest Group (SIG) of the International Forum on the Study of Itch (IFSI). Acta Derm Venereol 2015;95:261–5.

9. Stein BL, Oh ST, Berenzon D, et al. Polycythemia vera: an appraisal of the biology and management 10 years after the discovery of JAK2 V617F. J Clin Oncol 2015; 33:3953–60.

10. Scherber RM, Geyer HL, Mesa RA. Quality of life in MPN comes of age as a therapeutic target. Curr Hematol Malig Rep 2014;9:324–30.

11. Stein BL, Moliterno AR, Tiu RV. Polycythemia vera disease burden: contributing factors, impact on quality of life, and emerging treatment options. Ann Hematol 2014;93:1965–76.

12. Geyer H, Mesa RA. Assessing disease burden in patients with classic MPNs. Best Pract Res Clin Haematol 2014;27:107–19.

13. Lee G, Arcasoy MO. The clinical and laboratory evaluation of the patient with erythrocytosis. Eur J Intern Med 2015;26:297–302.

14. Tefferi A, Thiele J, Orazi A, et al. Proposals and rationale for revision of the World Health Organization diagnostic criteria for polycythemia vera, essential thrombocythemia, and primary myelofibrosis: recommendations from an ad hoc international expert panel. Blood 2007;110:1092–7.

15. Landolfi R, Marchioli R, Kutti J, et al. Efficacy and safety of low-dose aspirin in polycythemia vera. N Engl J Med 2004;350(2):114–24.

16. Tartaglia AP, Goldberg JD, Berk PD, et al. Adverse effects of antiaggregating platelet therapy in the treatment of polycythemia vera. Semin Hematol 1986; 23(3):172–6.

17. Marchioli R, Finazzi G, Landolfi R, et al. Vascular and neoplastic risk in a large cohort of patients with polycythemia vera. J Clin Oncol 2005;23(10):2224–32.

18. Bonicelli G, Abdulkarim K, Mounier M, et al. Leucocytosis and thrombosis at diagnosis are associated with poor survival in polycythaemia vera: a population-based study of 327 patients. Br J Haematol 2013;160(2):251–4.

19. Gangat N, Strand J, Li CY, et al. Leucocytosis in polycythaemia vera predicts both inferior survival and leukaemic transformation. Br J Haematol 2007;138(3): 354–8.

20. Marchioli R, Finazzi G, Specchia G, et al. Cardiovascular events and intensity of treatment in polycythemia vera. N Engl J Med 2013;368(1):22–33.

21. Vannucchi AM, Kiladjian JJ, Griesshammer M, et al. Ruxolitinib versus standard therapy for the treatment of polycythemia vera. N Engl J Med 2015;372(5): 426–35.

22. Kiladjian JJ, Cassinat B, Chevret S, et al. Pegylated interferon-alfa-2a induces complete hematologic and molecular responses with low toxicity in polycythemia vera. Blood 2008;112(8):3065–72.

23. Tefferi A, Guglielmelli P, Larson DR, et al. Long-term survival and blast transformation in molecularly annotated essential thrombocythemia, polycythemia vera, and myelofibrosis. Blood 2014;124(16):2507–13.

24. Kiladjian JJ, Chevret S, Dosquet C, et al. Treatment of polycythemia vera with hydroxyurea and pipobroman: final results of a randomized trial initiated in 1980. J Clin Oncol 2011;29:3907–13.

25. Carobbio A, Thiele J, Passamonti F, et al. Risk factors for arterial and venous thrombosis in WHO-defined essential thrombocythemia: an international study of 891 patients. Blood 2011;117:5857–9.

26. Passamonti F, Thiele J, Girodon F, et al. A prognostic model to predict survival in 867 World Health Organization-defined essential thrombocythemia at

diagnosis: a study by the International Working Group on myelofibrosis research and treatment. Blood 2012;120(6):1197–201.

27. Barbui T, Finazzi G, Carobbio A, et al. Development and validation of an international prognostic score of thrombosis in World Health Organization-essential thrombocythemia (IPSET-thrombosis). Blood 2012;120:5128–33.

28. Cortelazzo S, Finazzi G, Ruggeri M, et al. Hydroxyurea for patients with essential thrombocythemia and a high risk of thrombosis. N Engl J Med 1995;332:1132–6.

29. Harrison CN, Campbell PJ, Buck G, et al. Hydroxyurea compared with anagrelide in high-risk essential thrombocythemia. N Engl J Med 2005;353:33–45.

30. Iurlo A, Cattaneo D, Orofino N, et al. Anagrelide and mutational status in essential thrombocythemia. BioDrugs 2016;30(3):219–23.

31. Kiladjian JJ, Cassinat B, Turture P, et al. High molecular response rate of polycythemia vera patients treated with pegylated interferon alpha-2a. Blood 2006;108: 2037–40.

32. Verger E, Cassinat B, Chauveau A, et al. Clinical and molecular response to interferon-alpha therapy in essential thrombocythemia patients with CALR mutations. Blood 2015;126(24):2585–91.

33. Barbui T, Barosi G, Birgegard G, et al. Philadelphia-negative classical myeloproliferative neoplasms: critical concepts and management recommendations from European LeukemiaNet. J Clin Oncol 2011;29(6):761–70.

34. Pieri L, Pancrazzi A, Pacilli A, et al. JAK2V617F complete molecular remission in polycythemia vera/essential thrombocythemia patients treated with ruxolitinib. Blood 2015;125(21):3352–3.

35. Passamonti F, Rumi E, Pungolino E, et al. Life expectancy and prognostic factors for survival in patients with polycythemia vera and essential thrombocythemia. Am J Med 2004;117:755–61.

36. Cervantes F, Alvarez-Larran A, Talarn C, et al. Myelofibrosis with myeloid metaplasia following essential thrombocythaemia: actuarial probability, presenting characteristics and evolution in a series of 195 patients. Br J Haematol 2002; 118(3):786–90.

37. Wolanskyj AP, Schwager SM, McClure RF, et al. Essential thrombocythemia beyond the first decade: life expectancy, long-term complication rates, and prognostic factors. Mayo Clin Proc 2006;81(2):159–66.

38. Hobbs GS, Rampal RK. Clinical and molecular genetic characterization of myelofibrosis. Curr Opin Hematol 2015;22:177–83.

39. Spivak JL, Silver RT. The revised World Health Organization diagnostic criteria for polycythemia vera, essential thrombocytosis, and primary myelofibrosis: an alternative proposal. Blood 2008;112:231–9.

40. Harrison C, Kiladjian JJ, Al-Ali HK, et al. JAK inhibition with ruxolitinib versus best available therapy for myelofibrosis. N Engl J Med 2012;366(9):787–98.

41. Verstovsek S, Mesa RA, Gotlib J, et al. A double-blind, placebo-controlled trial of ruxolitinib for myelofibrosis. N Engl J Med 2012;366(9):799–807.

42. Cervantes F, Vannucchi AM, Kiladjian JJ, et al. Three-year efficacy, safety, and survival findings from COMFORT-II, a phase 3 study comparing ruxolitinib with best available therapy for myelofibrosis. Blood 2013;122(25):4047–53.

43. Saeidi K. Myeloproliferative neoplasms: current molecular biology and genetics. Crit Rev Oncol Hematol 2016;98:375–89.

Eosinophilia

Anna Kovalszki, MD[a],*, Peter F. Weller, MD[b]

KEYWORDS

- Eosinophilia • Asthma • Eosinophilic gastrointestinal disease • Drug allergy
- Parasitic disease • Hypereosinophilic syndromes

KEY POINTS

- Eosinophilia is an elevation in the total number of bloodstream eosinophils, can be transient or sustained, and can exist in milder versus more significant levels.
- Sustained and significant eosinophilia in the 1500 cells/μL or above range, without clear cause, should prompt evaluation.
- Processes known to cause modest eosinophilia include allergic disease, parasitic disease, drug allergy, and mastocytosis.
- More significant eosinophilia is often caused by drug allergy, aspirin exacerbated respiratory disease, sustained and significant atopic dermatitis, and some parasitic disorders.
- If no apparent cause of the eosinophilia is known and levels above 1500 cells/μL exist for greater than 1 month, an exhaustive search guided by clinical presentation should ensue.

INTRODUCTION

Eosinophilia represents an increased number of eosinophils in the tissues and/or blood. Although enumeration of tissue eosinophil numbers would require examination of biopsied tissues, blood eosinophil numbers are more readily and routinely measured. Hence, eosinophilia is often recognized based on an elevation of eosinophils in the blood. Absolute eosinophil counts exceeding 450 to 550 cells/μL, depending on laboratory standards, are reported as elevated. Percentages generally above 5% of the differential are regarded as elevated in most institutions, although the absolute count should be calculated before a determination of eosinophilia is made. This is done by multiplying the total white cell count by the percentage of eosinophils.

Eosinophils are bone marrow–derived cells of the granulocyte lineage. They have an approximate half-life of 8 to 18 hours in the bloodstream, and mostly reside in tissues[1] where they can persist for at least several weeks. Their functional roles are

Disclosure Statement: Neither author has relevant items to disclose for this article.
[a] Allergy and Inflammation, Beth Israel Deaconess Medical Center, Harvard Medical School, One Brookline Place Suite 623, Brookline, MA 02445, USA; [b] Allergy and Inflammation, Department of Medicine, Beth Israel Deaconess Medical Center, Harvard Medical School, CLS Building, Room 943, 330 Brookline Avenue, Boston, MA 02215, USA
* Corresponding author.
E-mail address: akovalsz@bidmc.harvard.edu

multifaceted and include antigen presentation; the release of lipid-derived, peptide, and cytokine mediators for acute and chronic inflammation; responses to helminth and parasite clearance through degranulation; and ongoing homeostatic immune responses. They can be part of the overall cellular milieu in malignant neoplasms and autoimmune conditions, and connective tissue disorders, and are also found in less well characterized entities as described elsewhere in this paper.

The approach to eosinophilia is largely based on clinical history. Often, a few aspects of a case alert the clinician as to the likely underlying cause of abnormally elevated eosinophils. However, at times, more significant investigations need to occur to more clearly define the cause of their presence and possible role in disease presentation.

Eosinophilia → 450 to 550 cells/μL in the blood stream

Allergic Sensitization

Mild eosinophilia is present often in patients with allergic disease (<1500 cells/μL will be used for the definition of mild, whereas hypereosinophilic syndromes, defined elsewhere in the article, are generally considered with sustained eosinophilia > 1500 cells/μL[2]). Allergic rhinitis and asthma often produce a mild eosinophilia. Atopic dermatitis may produce a more significant eosinophilia if affecting a large part of the body and if associated with significant atopy. Eosinophilic esophagitis as well as other eosinophilic gastrointestinal diseases can cause a mild peripheral eosinophilia.

Chronic sinusitis, especially of the polypoid variety seen in aspirin-exacerbated respiratory disease, produces a more robust eosinophilic response that can be in the mild to moderate range. Often these patients start with nasal allergies and asthma, but then develop abnormal arachidonic acid metabolizing cascades and hence have a more dramatic presentation both of their disease entity and of the eosinophilia.[3,4]

Allergic bronchopulmonary aspergillosis, related both to a fungus (Aspergillus) and to sensitization in an allergic/asthmatic host, can also produce varied and sometimes significant degrees of eosinophilia and also elevated total immunoglobulin (Ig)E.[5]

Chronic eosinophilic pneumonia often starts in a sensitized, asthmatic host. Although these patients may have milder peripheral eosinophilia at disease onset, they often have more moderate range eosinophilia later in the course. They also have bronchoalveolar lavage fluid that contains at least 40% eosinophils in up to 80% of cases.[6] This form of eosinophilic pneumonia can be premonitory to the later development of the eosinophilic vasculitis, eosinophilic granulomatosis with polyangiitis (EGPA), previously known as Churg-Strauss vasculitis.

Drug allergy can cause anywhere from mild to severe eosinophilia and often waxes quickly and wanes in a slower fashion; it can take months for eosinophilia from drug allergy to clear. There is usually, although not always, an associated drug rash of the diffuse/maculopapular variety. Patients can also present with asymptomatic eosinophilia owing to drugs, especially penicillins, cephalosporins, or quinolones.[7] Pulmonary infiltrates and peripheral eosinophilia have been associated with varied medications, including nonsteroidal antiinflammatory drugs, sulfa drugs, and nitrofurantoin.[7] Drug-induced diseases of other organs can also elicit tissue and blood eosinophilia (eg, drug-induced interstitial nephritis). **Box 1** summarizes causes of allergen-induced eosinophilia.

The drug rash with eosinophilia and systemic symptoms (DRESS) syndrome often produces significant eosinophil elevations in addition to liver function abnormalities, temperature dysregulation and lymphadenopathy. In reviews of 2 large,

---

Box 1
Causes of allergy associated eosinophilia

Mild degree of eosinophilia

- Allergic rhinitis
- Asthma
- Atopic dermatitis
- Eosinophilic esophagitis
- Drug allergy

Moderate to severe degree of eosinophilia

- Chronic sinusitis (especially polypoid and aspirin-exacerbated respiratory disease)
- Allergic bronchopulmonary aspergillosis
- Chronic eosinophilic pneumonia
- Drug allergy (drug rash with eosinophilia and systemic symptoms [DRESS] syndrome)

---

hospital-based cohorts of monitored drug allergies in Brazil and Malaysia, the DRESS syndrome was caused mainly by antibiotics, antiepileptics, antigout regimens, antiretrovirals, and nonsteroidal antiinflammatory drugs.[8,9] Stevens-Johnson syndrome and toxic epidermal necrolysis, severe and life-threating forms of drug allergy, do not usually produce eosinophilia, but rather neutrophilia and lymphocytopenia. **Box 2** lists pharmaceuticals commonly implicated in DRESS syndrome.

Parasite- and Infection-Related Eosinophilia

Tissue-dwelling helminths ("worms") are parasitic infections that often produce mild to moderate eosinophilia. Strongyloides infection is a common cause, whereas Giardia, a luminal parasite, does not cause eosinophilia. See **Box 3** for parasites that cause eosinophilia.

In the United States, parasites that can be contracted without any travel to foreign countries include strongyloides, trichinella, ascaris, hookworm, and visceral larva migrans (Toxocara from dogs/cats). In evaluating a patient for a possible helminthic etiology of the eosinophilia, testing for Strongyloides must be done because, unique among helminths, it can persist even decades after initial infection. Strongyloides can be asymptomatic or cause fleeting hives, dermatographism, angioedema, and/or abdominal pain. If a patient with undiagnosed Strongyloides infection receives

---

Box 2
Commonly implicated pharmaceuticals in drug rash with eosinophilia and systemic symptoms (DRESS) syndrome

Antibiotics: Penicillins, cephalosporins, dapsone, sulfa-based antibiotics

Xanthine oxidase inhibitor: Allopurinol

Antiepileptics: Carbamazepine, phenytoin, lamotrigine, valproic acid

Antiretrovirals: Nevirapine, efavirenz

Nonsteroidal antiinflammatory drugs: Ibuprofen

Box 3
Select parasitic infections that cause eosinophilia

Helminthic infections

Nematodes
- *Angiostrongyliasis costaricensis*
- Ascariasis
- Hookworm infection
- Strongyloidiasis
- Trichinellosis
- Visceral larva migrans
- Gnathostomiasis
- Cysticercosis
- Echinococcosis

Filariases
- Tropical pulmonary eosinophilia
- Loiasis
- Onchocerciasis

Flukes
- Schistosomiasis
- Fascioliasis
- Clonorchiasis
- Paragonimiasis
- Fasciolopsiasis

Protozoan infections

- *Isospora belli*

- *Dientamoeba fragilis*

- Sarcocystis

---

high-dose systemic corticosteroids, disseminated strongyloidiasis can ensue. This is sometimes associated with enteric bacterial sepsis and can be fatal.[10] The enzyme-linked immunosorbent antibody assay is a sensitive test for Strongyloides. Stool examinations for larvae are insensitive. Serologic or other evidence of ongoing strongyloidiasis merits ivermectin treatment, especially in an eosinophilic subject who may eventually be treated with corticosteroids.

Some fungi such as coccidioidomycosis (both acute and chronic), disseminated histoplasmosis (less commonly eosinophilic), and cryptococcosis (especially with central nervous system infections) also have been associated with eosinophilia. Coccidioides is found in the Southwestern United States as well as Mexico, and Central and South Americas. Histoplasma contaminates bird and bat droppings, so cave exploring and living in areas with heavy pigeon populations can lead to significant exposures. Cryptococcus is found in soil throughout the world. These infections are often more significant and disseminated in immunocompromised hosts.

The retrovirus, human T-cell lymphocytic virus-1, is one of the few viruses associated with eosinophilia. It is prevalent in Japan, Africa, the Caribbean Islands, and South America, and newly found in Eastern Europe and the Middle East.[11] Human immunodeficiency virus-1–infected patients may have eosinophilia not directly related to the infection but from secondary phenomena (drug allergy, eosinophilic folliculitis[12]).

In contrast with the "rule" that only helminthic parasites may elicit eosinophilia, there are 3 protozoa that can cause peripheral eosinophilia. *Isospora belli* and *Dientamoeba fragilis*,[13] both intestinal protozoa, and Sarcocystitis, a rare tissue-dwelling protozoa, are found only in those with exposures in areas of Southeast Asia.

Autoimmune Disease

EGPA, previously known as Churg-Strauss syndrome, arises usually in an atopic individual and produces varying degrees of sinus disease, lung disease, and kidney disease and can cause mononeuritis multiplex and vascular disease as well. EGPA is associated with significant eosinophilia, increased inflammatory markers, and tissue eosinophilia in affected areas. It carries in its differential diagnosis and shares many aspects with hypereosinophilic syndromes (discussed elsewhere in this article). The vasculitis is often identified late in the course of the disease, especially if the kidney is not involved. EGPA with eosinophilia and predominantly nonhemorrhagic lung manifestations has a significantly lower prevalence of antineutrophil cytoplasmic antibody positivity (perinuclear antineutrophil cytoplasmic antibody) than EGPA with renal involvement, so antineutrophil cytoplasmic antibody tests do not exclude EGPA disease.[14] EGPA produces both eosinophilia and symptoms out of proportion to usual allergic complications, with sinus, lung, and other organ involvement. In the initial evaluation of patients with possible EGPA, the latest consensus recommendations from 2015 suggest serologic testing for toxocariasis and human immunodeficiency virus, specific IgE and IgG for *Aspergillus* spp., search for *Aspergillus* spp. in sputum and/or bronchoalveolar lavage fluid (to evaluate for allergic bronchopulmonary aspergillosis), tryptase, and vitamin B_{12} levels (to evaluate for myeloproliferative hypereosinophilic syndrome), peripheral blood smear (looking for dysplastic eosinophils or blasts suggestive of primary eosinophilic bone marrow process), and chest computed tomography scan (to evaluate for lung involvement). Additional workup should be guided by presentation. Referral for more specific evaluation by a qualified rheumatologist or immunologist at a center that treats patients with vasculitis is recommended given the elusive nature of EGPA as well as clinical implications if it is undertreated.[15] **Fig. 1** is a characteristic computed tomography scan of the chest done to evaluate a patient with EGPA treated at our institution.

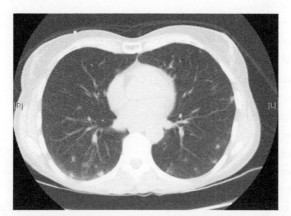

Fig. 1. Computed tomography (CT) scan of the chest of a patient with eosinophilic granulomatosis with polyangiitis. Areas of diffuse ground glass opacities and consolidations in both right and left lungs. This finding is characteristic of how small-vessel vasculitides affect the lungs. (Patient of Anna Kovalszki, MD; CT scan taken at Beth Israel Deaconess Medical Center, Boston, MA.)

Connective tissue/autoimmune diseases to a variable extent can be associated with peripheral eosinophilia. Eosinophils are present as part of the overall inflammatory milieu, even if they are not the cell types implicated in disease pathogenesis necessarily. The degree of eosinophilia is not well-established in these cases. For example, in a retrospective analysis, mild degrees of eosinophilia were felt to be related to certain rheumatic disorders, but the authors felt that treatment with nonsteroidal antiinflammatory drugs and corticosteroids confounded the frequency of eosinophilia found.[16] In a case report of severe rheumatoid arthritis, up to 24,000 eosinophils/mm³ were seen.[17]

In inflammatory bowel diseases, blood eosinophil levels can be elevated, yet the roles of eosinophils in gastrointestinal diseases are still being elucidated. For instance, levels of the eosinophil-recruiting chemokine, eotaxin-1, in the tissues were correlated with tissue eosinophilia of ulcerative colitis patients in the active disease state.[18] In sarcoidosis, mild peripheral eosinophilia was common, even without other atopic disease present in a retrospective cohort of sarcoid patients.[19] In IgG4-related disease, a relatively newly recognized entity known to produce tissue infiltration and tumorlike destruction of certain glands, organs, and lymph nodes, blood eosinophilia can be present in about 25% and both IgE elevations and mild to moderate blood eosinophilia occurred in an atopy-independent fashion.[20]

Often with these disorders (listed in **Box 4**), an exhaustive search is usually done if the eosinophilia is persistent and marked. Even though these disorders can be associated with eosinophilia to some degree, often patients are on many medications and more common reasons for eosinophilia such as drug allergy need to be ruled out.

Primary Eosinophilia

Hypereosinophilic syndromes (idiopathic, myeloproliferative variant, and lymphocytic variant) are a group of disorders in which eosinophilia is always present and can be

---

Box 4
Eosinophilia associated with connective tissue, rheumatologic, and autoimmune disease

- Eosinophilic fasciitis
- Eosinophilic granulomatosis with polyangiitis (Churg-Strauss vasculitis)
- Dermatomyositis
- Severe rheumatoid arthritis
- Progressive systemic sclerosis
- Sjögren syndrome
- Thromboangiitis obliterans with eosinophilia of the temporal arteries
- Granulomatosis with polyangiitis (Wegener syndrome)
- Systemic lupus erythematosus
- Behçet syndrome
- IgG4-related disease
- Inflammatory bowel disease
- Sarcoidosis
- Bullous pemphigoid
- Dermatitis herpetiformis (celiac disease)

moderate to severe. The underlying cause can have a defined etiology or be completely idiopathic. Affected organs can include lungs, skin, heart, blood vessels, sinuses, kidneys, and brain. Patients with idiopathic disease can present asymptomatically or with ongoing fatigue, myalgias, weakness, and general malaise. Workup can be unrevealing except for the eosinophilia, which may be recalcitrant even to corticosteroid treatment.

Often, patients with a lymphocytic variant have diffuse skin manifestations (pruritus, ongoing erythema, rash). They often have a CD3⁻ CD4⁺ population of T cells and/or abnormal T-cell receptor clonality. They are at risk for developing T-cell lymphomas. They can be especially difficult to manage with ongoing monitoring for neoplasm development and ongoing need for oral corticosteroids (with response) and other disease-modifying drugs.[21]

Patients with a myeloproliferative variant often have heart disease or thrombotic complications (endomyocardial inflammation and stroke), splenomegaly, elevated tryptase level, elevated lactate dehydrogenase, and increased vitamin B_{12} level. They can have FIP1L1-PDGFRA and other related chromosomal mutations, and are responsive to imatinib. Imatinib can be useful in some who lack the FIP1L1-PDGFRA mutation if they have myeloproliferative features.[22]

Episodic angioedema associated with eosinophilia (Gleich syndrome[23]) is associated with marked episodic eosinophilia, angioedema, urticaria, pruritus, fever, weight gain, and often an elevated IgM level. These patients have an underlying immune dyscrasia driving their presentation, with an elevation in eosinophils associated with antecedent increases in cytokine interleukin-5 levels. Many also have an aberrant CD3⁻ CD4⁺ T-cell population and T-cell receptor clonality as well.[24]

In 25% of patients with mastocytosis, there is an associated eosinophilia, usually in the mild to moderate range. There is thought to be significant cross-talk between mast cells and eosinophils.[25] Most patients have a mutation (D816V) in the c-KIT gene. Systemic mastocytosis patients with D816VKIT mutations have concurrently presented with FIP1L1-PDGFRA mutations and chronic eosinophilic leukemia, although this is a rare event. Bone marrow biopsy in mastocytosis and chronic eosinophilic leukemia exhibit some common pathologic features, such as CD25 expression on mast cells and spindle shaped mast cell morphology.[26]

Box 5 summarizes clinical entities associated with primary eosinophil burden and likely disease-related pathogenesis.

Box 5
Primary eosinophilias

Idiopathic hypereosinophilic syndrome: sustained peripheral eosinophilia at greater than 1500 cells/μL with associated end-organ damage.

Lymphoproliferative hypereosinophilic syndrome: sustained peripheral eosinophilia at greater than 1500 cell/μL, often associated with rash, aberrant T-cell immunophenotypic profile, often steroid responsive.

Myeloproliferative hypereosinophilic syndrome: sustained peripheral eosinophilia at greater than 1500 cell/μL, often features of splenomegaly, heart related complications, and thrombosis. Can have associated FIP1L1-PDGFRA and other mutations and are often steroid resistant. Patients can be considered to have a diagnosis of chronic eosinophilic leukemia.

Episodic eosinophilia associated with angioedema (G syndrome): cyclical fevers, swelling, hives, pruritus, marked eosinophilia, and IgM elevation. Aberrant T-cell phenotypes often associated.

Malignancy-Related Eosinophilia

There are eosinophil-derived malignancies (acute and chronic eosinophilic leukemia) and malignancies in which eosinophils are increased as part of the overall cellular milieu. **Box 6** lists malignancies associated with eosinophilia.

Immunodeficiency-Related Eosinophilia

Autosomal-dominant hyper-IgE syndrome (Job syndrome), with recurrent abscesses, lung infections, and severe eczema, is associated with eosinophilia. Wiskott-Aldrich syndrome, with eczema, thrombocytopenia, and recurrent infections in an X-linked fashion, also causes peripheral and tissue eosinophilia. Adenosine deaminase severe combined immunodeficiency also has eosinophilic associations. Atopy is a common feature in this entity in addition to severe immunodeficiency with recurrent infections starting in infancy. Omenn syndrome causes profound peripheral eosinophilia, IgE elevation, and abnormally elevated T cells as well as autoimmunity and an erythrodermic rash. Patients are often discovered in newborn screening and undergo transplantation.[27]

Miscellaneous Entities Associated with Eosinophilia

Rejection of transplanted solid organs including liver, pancreas, kidney, and heart have been associated with peripheral and organ-specific eosinophilia. The eosinophilia can be moderate to severe.[28]

Chronic graft-versus-host disease after hematopoietic stem cell transplantation has also caused peripheral eosinophilia. Level of skin involvement and severity of graft-versus-host disease could not be reliably predicted based on the presence of eosinophilia in 1 cohort of patients.[29]

Kimura disease, a disease of mostly Asian males, is defined as masslike lymph node or subcutaneous tissue swelling mainly in the head and neck, peripheral eosinophilia, IgE elevation, and eosinophilic pathologic infiltrates with follicular hyperplasia and proliferation of postcapillary venules in biopsies. Surgical excision and steroid therapy is often used.[30]

Epithelioid hemangioma, also known as angiolymphoid hyperplasia with eosinophilia, also most often affects the head and neck, especially on and around the auricles. It is seen in all races and both sexes, affects the dermis or epidermis, and is thought of as a benign vascular proliferative disease. Excision and laser therapy

---

Box 6
Malignancy-associated eosinophilia

Blood-related neoplasms

- Acute or chronic eosinophilic leukemia
- Lymphoma (T cell and Hodgkin)
- Chronic myelomonocytic leukemia

Solid organ–associated neoplasms

- Adenocarcinomas of the gastrointestinal tract (gastric, colorectal)
- Lung cancer
- Squamous epithelium related cancers (cervix, vagina, penis, skin, nasopharynx, bladder)
- Thyroid cancer

Box 7
Entities that can be associated with eosinophilia

- Rejection of a transplanted solid organ
- Graft-versus-host disease after hematopoietic stem cell transplantation
- Kimura disease and epithelioid hemangioma
- Eosinophilia-myalgia syndrome/toxic oil syndrome
- Adrenal insufficiency
- Irritation of serosal surfaces
- Cholesterol embolus

---

seem to be the most often used treatment modalities, often undertaken for cosmetic reasons.[31] Peripheral eosinophilia is variable and IgE elevation is not common.

Historical syndromes caused by toxic ingestions included the eosinophilia–myalgia syndrome and the toxic oil syndrome. Contaminated (impure) L-tryptophan caused the eosinophilia–myalgia syndrome in 1989 in the United States, characterized by myalgias, skin induration, and eosinophilia. This occurred from a single source of L-tryptophan, which has since been banned by the US Food and Drug Administration. Analine-denatured cooking grade oils produced by a specific refinery in Seville, Spain, in 1981 caused the toxic oil syndrome. Symptoms were myalgias, eosinophilia, and pulmonary infiltrates. Both of these episodes caused significant morbidity and mortality. These are historical events, but could in theory occur again with other manufactured ingestible items.[32] The specific mechanisms and subtypes of contaminants responsible for the disorders were never fully elucidated.

Eosinophils are sensitive even to endogenous corticosteroid production. Therefore, absence of corticosteroids can induce a peripheral eosinophilia. Such hypoadrenalism may happen in Addison disease or adrenal hemorrhage.

Irritation of serosal surfaces can cause peripheral eosinophilia. Peritoneal dialysis catheters can produce peritoneal eosinophilia, which can in turn be detected peripherally.

Cholesterol embolization, owing to instrumentation or other trauma to the aorta, can cause purplish discoloration of toes, livedo reticularis, renal disease, elevated inflammatory markers, and hypocomplementemia, along with mild to moderate transient eosinophilia, which can provide a diagnostic clue.[33] **Box 7** lists miscellaneous entities that can be associated with eosinophilia.

SUMMARY

Eosinophilia, greater than 450 to 500 eosinophils/μL in peripheral blood, is a hallmark of or a related finding in many allergic, infectious, autoimmune, idiopathic, malignant, and miscellaneous clinical scenarios. The clinical history is often the most important clue in discovering a pathway by which the patient is possibly affected by eosinophilia. Tailored evaluation based on scenario, including allergy testing, laboratory testing, imaging, and pathologic biopsy of affected areas can be useful in confirming a diagnosis. A broad differential diagnosis is often narrowed based on careful observation and clinical evaluation. Should findings point to specific areas, referral to appropriate specialists may be warranted. This referral spectrum in the case of eosinophilia is broad and often related to which organ system is involved.

REFERENCES

1. Kovalszki A, Sheikh J, Weller PF. Eosinophils and Eosinophilia. In: Rich RR, editor. Clinical immunology principles and practice. 4th edition. London: Elsevier Saunders; 2013. p. 298–309.

2. Ogbogu PU, Bochner BS, Butterfield JH, et al. Hypereosinophilic syndrome: a multicenter, retrospective analysis of clinical characteristics and response to therapy. J Allergy Clin Immunol 2009;124(6):1319–25.e3.

3. Stevens WW, Ocampo CJ, Berdnikovs S, et al. Cytokines in chronic rhinosinusitis. role in eosinophilia and aspirin-exacerbated respiratory disease. Am J Respir Crit Care Med 2015;192(6):682–94.

4. Laidlaw TM, Boyce JA. Aspirin-exacerbated respiratory disease–new prime suspects. N Engl J Med 2016;374(5):484–8.

5. Saxena S, Madan T, Shah A, et al. Association of polymorphisms in the collagen region of SP-A2 with increased levels of total IgE antibodies and eosinophilia in patients with allergic bronchopulmonary aspergillosis. J Allergy Clin Immunol 2003;111(5):1001–7.

6. Akuthota P, Weller PF. Eosinophilic pneumonias. Clin Microbiol Rev 2012;25(4): 649–60.

7. Nutman TB. Evaluation and differential diagnosis of marked, persistent eosinophilia. Immunol Allergy Clin North Am 2007;27(3):529–49.

8. Grando LR, Schmitt TA, Bakos RM. Severe cutaneous reactions to drugs in the setting of a general hospital. An Bras Dermatol 2014;89(5):758–62.

9. Choon SE, Lai NM. An epidemiological and clinical analysis of cutaneous adverse drug reactions seen in a tertiary hospital in Johor, Malaysia. Indian J Dermatol Venereol Leprol 2012;78(6):734–9.

10. Newberry AM, Williams DN, Stauffer WM, et al. Strongyloides hyperinfection presenting as acute respiratory failure and gram-negative sepsis. Chest 2005; 128(5):3681–4.

11. Stienlauf S, Yahalom V, Schwartz E, et al. Epidemiology of human T-cell lymphotropic virus type 1 infection in blood donors, Israel. Emerg Infect Dis 2009;15(7): 1116–8.

12. Rane SR, Agrawal PB, Kadgi NV, et al. Histopathological study of cutaneous manifestations in HIV and AIDS patients. Int J Dermatol 2014;53(6):746–51.

13. Gray TJ, Kwan YL, Phan T, et al. Dientamoeba fragilis: a family cluster of disease associated with marked peripheral eosinophilia. Clin Infect Dis 2013;57(6):845–8.

14. Sinico RA, Di Toma L, Maggiore U, et al. Prevalence and clinical significance of antineutrophil cytoplasmic antibodies in Churg-Strauss syndrome. Arthritis Rheum 2005;52(9):2926–35.

15. Groh M, Pagnoux C, Baldini C, et al. Eosinophilic granulomatosis with polyangiitis (Churg-Strauss) (EGPA) Consensus Task Force recommendations for evaluation and management. Eur J Intern Med 2015;26(7):545–53.

16. Kargili A, Bavbek N, Kaya A, et al. Eosinophilia in rheumatologic diseases: a prospective study of 1000 cases. Rheumatol Int 2004;24(6):321–4.

17. Rosenstein RK, Panush RS, Kramer N, et al. Hypereosinophilia and seroconversion of rheumatoid arthritis. Clin Rheumatol 2014;33(11):1685–8.

18. Adar T, Shteingart S, Ben-Ya'acov A, et al. The importance of intestinal eotaxin-1 in inflammatory bowel disease: New insights and possible therapeutic implications. Dig Dis Sci 2016;61(7):1915–24.

19. Takahashi A, Konno S, Hatanaka K, et al. A case of sarcoidosis with eosinophilia in peripheral blood and bronchoalveolar lavage fluid. Respir Med Case Rep 2013;8:43–6.
20. Della Torre E, Mattoo H, Mahajan VS, et al. Prevalence of atopy, eosinophilia, and IgE elevation in IgG4-related disease. Allergy 2014;69(2):269–72.
21. Lefevre G, Copin MC, Staumont-Sallé D, et al. The lymphoid variant of hypereosinophilic syndrome: study of 21 patients with CD3-CD4+ aberrant T-cell phenotype. Medicine (Baltimore) 2014;93(17):255–66.
22. Khoury P, Desmond R, Pabon A, et al. Clinical features predict responsiveness to imatinib in platelet-derived growth factor receptor-alpha-negative hypereosinophilic syndrome. Allergy 2016;71(6):803–10.
23. Gleich GJ, Schroeter AL, Marcoux JP, et al. Episodic angioedema associated with eosinophilia. N Engl J Med 1984;310(25):1621–6.
24. Khoury P, Herold J, Alpaugh A, et al. Episodic angioedema with eosinophilia (Gleich syndrome) is a multilineage cell cycling disorder. Haematologica 2015; 100(3):300–7.
25. Kovalszki A, Weller PF. Eosinophilia in mast cell disease. Immunol Allergy Clin North Am 2014;34(2):357–64.
26. Gotlib J, Akin C. Mast cells and eosinophils in mastocytosis, chronic eosinophilic leukemia, and non-clonal disorders. Semin Hematol 2012;49(2):128–37.
27. Williams KW, Milner JD, Freeman AF. Eosinophilia associated with disorders of immune deficiency or immune dysregulation. Immunol Allergy Clin North Am 2015;35(3):523–44.
28. Weir MR, Bartlett ST, Drachenberg CB. Eosinophilia as an early indicator of pancreatic allograft rejection. Clin Transplant 2012;26(2):238–41.
29. Mortensen KB, Gerds TA, Bjerrum OW, et al. The prevalence and prognostic value of concomitant eosinophilia in chronic graft-versus-host disease after allogeneic stem cell transplantation. Leuk Res 2014;38(3):334–9.
30. Kar IB, Sethi AK. Kimura's disease: report of a case & review of literature. J Maxillofac Oral Surg 2013;12(1):109–12.
31. Adler BL, Krausz AE, Minuti A, et al. Epidemiology and treatment of angiolymphoid hyperplasia with eosinophilia (ALHE): A systematic review. J Am Acad Dermatol 2016;74(3):506–12.e11.
32. Gelpi E, de la Paz MP, Terracini B, et al. The Spanish toxic oil syndrome 20 years after its onset: a multidisciplinary review of scientific knowledge. Environ Health Perspect 2002;110(5):457–64.
33. Kasinath BS, Lewis EJ. Eosinophilia as a clue to the diagnosis of atheroembolic renal disease. Arch Intern Med 1987;147(8):1384–5.

Thrombosis, Hypercoagulable States, and Anticoagulants

Marie A. Hollenhorst, MD, PhD[a], Elisabeth M. Battinelli, MD, PhD[b],*

KEYWORDS

- Venous thromboembolism • Pulmonary embolism • Deep venous thrombosis
- Thrombophilia • Anticoagulation

KEY POINTS

- Thrombophilias are inherited or acquired derangements of secondary hemostasis that confer an increased risk of VTE.
- The most common inherited thrombophilias are factor V Leiden and the prothrombin gene mutation.
- The goal of the history and physical examination in a patient with suspected VTE is to determine the pretest probability of VTE, which should guide the decision of whether to pursue further work-up with D dimer or imaging.
- Testing for hypercoagulable disorders should be pursued only in patients with VTE who have an increased risk for an underlying hypercoagulable disorder.
- DOACs are the preferred medications for VTE treatment except in patients who are pregnant, have active cancer, antiphospholipid antibody syndrome, severe renal insufficiency, or prosthetic heart valves.

INTRODUCTION

Venous thromboemboli (VTE) are major causes of morbidity and mortality. The two most common types of VTE, deep venous thrombosis (DVT) and pulmonary embolism (PE), have an estimated incidence of 900,000 and mortality of 100,000 to 180,000 in the United States each year.[1,2] This article reviews the pathophysiology, diagnosis, and management of venous thromboembolic disease, with an emphasis on hypercoagulable states and direct oral anticoagulants (DOACs).

Disclosure statement: The authors have nothing to disclose.

[a] Internal Medicine, Brigham and Women's Hospital, 75 Francis Street, Boston, MA 02115, USA;
[b] Division of Hematology, Brigham and Women's Hospital, 75 Francis Street, Boston, MA 02115, USA
* Corresponding author.
E-mail address: ebattinelli@partners.org

PATHOPHYSIOLOGY

Venous thrombosis results from derangements of the hemostatic mechanism, which involves interactions between the vascular endothelium, platelets, and coagulation proteins. There are two components of hemostasis: primary hemostasis, which is initiated when endothelial injury results in exposure of subendothelial matrix components, triggering platelet adherence, activation, and aggregation; and secondary hemostasis, the coagulation cascade–dependent deposition of fibrin that forms a mesh that stabilizes the platelet plug. The coagulation cascade involves a series of proenzymes that are serially activated in a process that culminates in the formation of fibrin (**Fig. 1**). Predisposing factors to venous thrombosis are describe by Virchow's triad: (1) venous stasis, (2) hypercoagulability (inherited or acquired abnormality of secondary hemostasis), and (3) vascular injury.

There are several endogenous negative regulators of the coagulation cascade, including protein C, protein S, and antithrombin (AT) III. Thrombin converts protein C to activated protein C (APC). APC acts in concert with protein S to proteolytically inactivate factors Va and VIIIa, providing a negative feedback loop that limits thrombin production. AT III binds to and inactivates thrombin, factor Xa, and other clotting cascade proteases.

TYPES OF THROMBOSIS

DVT is clotting of blood in a deep vein, most commonly of the lower extremity. Lower extremity DVTs are classified as distal if the thrombi are confined to deep calf veins, and proximal if there is thrombosis in the popliteal or more proximal veins (femoral or iliac). Proximal DVTs are at higher risk of progression to PE than distal DVTs. Upper extremity DVT most commonly occurs as a result of endothelial trauma caused by placement of intravenous catheters.

Most commonly, a PE develops when a DVT detaches from its site of origin and travels through progressively larger veins, eventually reaching the right side of the heart and then lodging in the pulmonary artery or one of its branches.

DVT and PE are the most common venous thrombotic conditions and the most common presenting manifestations of hypercoagulable states. There are a variety of less common venous thrombotic presentations that occur with increased frequency in certain hypercoagulable states (**Tables 1** and **2**).

HYPERCOAGULABLE STATES
Inherited Thrombophilia

The most common cause of inherited thrombophilia is the factor V Leiden mutation, and the second most common cause is the prothrombin gene mutation (see **Table 1**). Together these account for about half of the inherited thrombophilias. The remainder is mostly caused by defects of AT, protein S, and protein C.

A single point mutation in the factor V gene results in the production of factor V Leiden, which is resistant to cleavage by protein C. Risk of thrombosis is increased in factor V Leiden heterozygotes, and is even higher in homozygotes (see **Table 1**). The most common clinical manifestation in patients with factor V Leiden is DVT with or without PE, but these patients are also at increased risk for other venous thromboses, such as cerebral, mesenteric, and portal vein. Testing for factor V Leiden is done either via genetic testing of peripheral blood to look for the causative mutation, or via functional APC resistance assays.

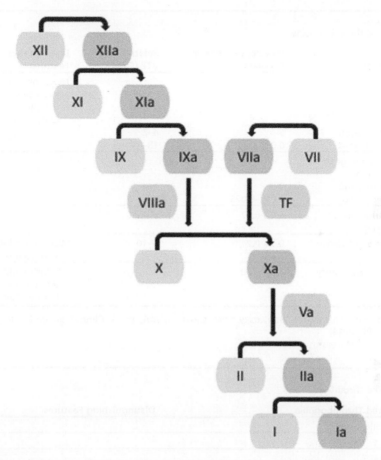

Fig. 1. Coagulation cascade. The pathway is initiated via one of two pathways, intrinsic and extrinsic, which each result in the conversion of factor X to its activated form Xa. The intrinsic pathway is activated by contact with negatively charged surfaces, and involves serial activation of factors XII, XI, and IX. Factors IXa, VIIIa, and X, in the presence of calcium and phospholipid, then form the tenase complex, which activates factor X to Xa. The extrinsic pathway is activated by contact with tissue factor (TF) that is exposed by endothelial damage. Factor VII is activated by TF to factor VIIa, which in complex with TF activates factor X to Xa. The intrinsic and extrinsic pathways each converge on the common pathway, which involves binding of factor Xa to factor Va in the presence of calcium and phospholipid to form the prothrombinase complex, which converts prothrombin (factor II) to thrombin (IIa). Thrombin then cleaves fibrinogen (factor I) to fibrin (factor Ia).

Prothrombin G20210A is a mutation in the 3′ untranslated region of the prothrombin gene that results in supranormal plasma levels of prothrombin. Prothrombin G20210A carriers are at increased risk for DVT/PE, abdominal vein thrombosis, and cerebral vein thrombosis. Testing for prothrombin G20210A is done via polymerase chain reaction–based genomic assay.

AT deficiency leads to a hypercoagulable state because of decreased anticoagulant activity of AT. Hereditary AT deficiency is a rare autosomal-dominant condition with variable penetrance. A variety of genetic alterations can lead to this condition, which

Table 1
Inherited thrombophilias

Inherited Thrombophilia	Prevalence: General Population (%)	Relative Risk VTE (OR)	Distinguishing Features
Factor V Leiden mutation			Most common inherited thrombophilia in Caucasians
Heterozygous	5	4–7	
Homozygous	0.065–0.2	18–80	
Prothrombin gene mutation			
Heterozygous	2–3	2–4	
Homozygous	0.012–0.025	NA	
Antithrombin deficiency	0.02–0.17	10–20	
Protein S deficiency	0.16–0.21	5–10	Warfarin-induced skin necrosis
Protein C deficiency	0.14–0.50	7	Warfarin-induced skin necrosis, Purpura fulminans

Adapted from Murray MF, Babyatsky MW, Giovanni MA, et al. Clinical genomics. New York: McGraw Hill, 2014.

Table 2
Acquired thrombophilias

Acquired Thrombophilia	Distinguishing Features
Immobilization	
Surgery	
Trauma	
Medications	
Oral contraceptives	
Hormone-replacement therapy	
Tamoxifen	
Lenalidomide	
Malignancy	Migratory superficial thrombophlebitis (Trousseau syndrome)
Smoking	
Pregnancy	
Antiphospholipid antibody syndrome	Arterial thrombosis Recurrent fetal loss Elevated partial thromboplastin time Thrombocytopenia
Myeloproliferative disorders	Hepatic and portal vein thrombosis
Polycythemia vera	Polycythemia
Essential thrombocythemia	Thrombocythemia
Paroxysmal nocturnal hemoglobinuria	Hepatic and portal vein thrombosis Pancytopenia Hemolysis

can arise either from deficiency of AT or dysfunctional protein. There are also several acquired conditions that can lead to AT deficiency, including asparaginase treatment, liver disease, and nephrotic syndrome. The most common manifestation of AT deficiency is DVT/PE. These patients are also at risk for abdominal vein thrombosis. Some patients exhibit heparin resistance, such that the partial thromboplastin time (PTT) is not prolonged when heparin is administered; these patients may benefit from AT-replacement therapy. Testing for AT deficiency is done using the AT-heparin cofactor assay, which measures the ability of heparin to bind to a coagulation factor that requires AT activity.

Protein C and S deficiencies can be caused by low levels of these proteins, or by decreased functional activity of the enzymes. Homozygous or compound heterozygous protein C deficiency typically presents in infancy with purpura fulminans. Heterozygous protein C and S deficiencies can present in teenagers and adults with VTE and as warfarin-induced skin necrosis. Testing for protein C and S deficiency using functional assays is the preferred approach.

Acquired Thrombophilia

There are many acquired risk factors for VTE (see **Table 2**). A key risk factor for VTE is immobilization and consequent venous stasis. Important causes of immobility include medical illness, surgery, and extended travel.[3] Several medications can lead to a hypercoagulable state, most notably oral contraceptives. Pregnant women are at increased risk of thrombosis because of stasis as a result of the gravid uterus leading to decreased venous return, and of hypercoagulability in the setting of pregnancy.

The antiphospholipid antibody syndrome (APLS) is an acquired thrombophilia characterized by vascular thromboses and/or pregnancy morbidity in the presence of antiphospholipid antibodies (**Table 3**).

Patients with chronic myeloproliferative neoplasms, especially essential thrombocythemia and polycythemia vera, are at increased risk for venous and arterial thromboembolic disease. Hepatic or portal vein thrombosis should raise the consideration of a myeloproliferative neoplasm, especially in a patient with polycythemia or thrombocytosis.

Paroxysmal nocturnal hemoglobinuria leads to an increased risk of venous thrombosis, especially abdominal and cerebral. This disorder is an acquired clonal bone marrow stem cell disorder that typically presents with pancytopenia and intravascular hemolysis.

VENOUS THROMBOEMBOLI DIAGNOSIS

There has been substantial work done to develop algorithms for VTE diagnosis that allow for minimization of unnecessary testing while maintaining high sensitivity for the diagnosis. The goal of the history and physical examination of a patient with suspected PE or DVT is to establish the pretest probability that the patient has one or both of these disorders. This is critical in stratifying patients into different risk groups to determine what further diagnostic testing should be pursued.

History

The typical symptoms of DVT include swelling, erythema, and/or pain of the affected extremity. The most common presenting symptom of PE is dyspnea, which is usually rapid in onset, within seconds or minutes.[4] Other common symptoms include pleuritic pain, cough, orthopnea, wheezing, and hemoptysis. About half of patients with PE also present with symptoms suggestive of lower extremity DVT.

| Table 3 |
| Antiphospholipid antibody syndrome diagnosis |

| **When to Suspect Antiphospholipid Antibody Syndrome** |
| Unexplained thrombotic events, especially arterial thromboses |
| Pregnancy morbidity |
| Unexplained thrombocytopenia or prolonged partial thromboplastin time |

| **Revised Sapporo Criteria** |
| **Definite APLS Is Considered if a Patient Meets at Least One Clinical and One Laboratory Criterion** |

Clinical	Presence of either vascular thrombosis or pregnancy morbidity	Vascular thrombosis One or more confirmed episodes of venous, arterial, or small vessel thromboses Pregnancy morbidity Unexplained fetal death at ≥10 wk gestation Premature birth at <34 wk of gestation Three or more unexplained <10 wk gestation
Laboratory	Presence of antiphospholipid antibodies on two or more occasions, at least 12 wk apart no more than 5 y preceding clinical manifestations	Laboratory studies indicative of antiphospholipid antibodies Lupus anticoagulant Anticardiolipin antibody (IgG and/or IgM) Anti-β-2-glycoprotein-I antibody (IgG and/or IgM)

Patients should be asked about recent hospitalizations, surgeries, or extended travel. A thorough past medical and medication history should be elicited to determine if the patient has any underlying health condition or medications that may predispose to VTE. If the patient has had any prior thrombosis, he or she should be questioned about any risk factors that may have been present at the time of the prior clot. An obstetric history should be obtained, because a history of spontaneous abortion could raise suspicion for APLS or an inherited thrombophilia. The status of routine cancer screening should be ascertained, as should any history of malignancy, and any symptoms suggestive of undiagnosed malignancy (fatigue, loss of appetite, or weight loss). Patients should also be questioned about family history of VTE or malignancy.

Physical Examination

Patients with DVT may have unilateral extremity swelling, erythema, and tenderness to deep palpation. The thrombosed vein may be evident as a palpable cord. The most common physical examination finding for PE is tachypnea. Other common signs include tachycardia, hypoxia, and decreased breath sounds. Patients with massive PE can present with hypotension, bradycardia, or pulselessness.

Differential Diagnosis

Important alternate diagnoses to consider in a patient with suspected DVT include cellulitis, superficial thrombophlebitis, ruptured Baker cyst, calf muscle tear, drug-induced lower extremity edema, and lymphedema. The differential diagnosis for PE includes asthma, chronic obstructive pulmonary disease, pneumothorax, pneumonia, pulmonary edema, pericarditis, pleuritis, and myocardial ischemia.

Pretest Probability

Several scoring systems have been developed to determine the pretest probability that a patient has VTE based on history and examination, including the Wells scores for DVT and PE (**Tables 4** and **5**).[5–8] For patients with signs and symptoms concerning for PE who are deemed low risk by the Wells score, the PE Rule-Out Criteria (PERC; **Table 6**) is used to determine if further evaluation with a D dimer assay is warranted.[9–12]

D Dimer

High-sensitivity enzyme-linked immunosorbent plasma D dimer tests measure the level of fibrin breakdown. They are highly sensitive but not very specific for VTE, and therefore are useful for ruling out VTE in patients with low pretest probability of clot. Current data support using age-adjusted D dimer cutoff values in patients greater than 50 years old (age $\times$ 10 ng/mL) for evaluation of PE. For DVT evaluation, a cutoff value of 500 ng/mL is used regardless of age.[13,14]

Imaging Studies

The imaging study of choice for evaluation of suspected DVT is venous ultrasonography. The diagnostic finding for DVT is loss of compressibility of the vein when pressure is applied with the ultrasound transducer. Computed tomography (CT) with intravenous contrast and magnetic resonance venography are used as alternatives or adjunctives to ultrasound.

PE protocol CT (PE-CT) with intravenous contrast is the diagnostic test of choice for diagnosis of PE. Ventilation perfusion scans are used as an alternative

Table 4 Wells score for DVT	
Clinical Feature	**Score**
Active cancer (treatment ongoing or within the previous 6 mo or palliative)	1
Paralysis, paresis, or recent plaster immobilization of the lower extremities	1
Recently bedridden for more than 3 d or major surgery, within 4 wk	1
Localized tenderness along the distribution of the deep venous system	1
Entire leg swollen	1
Calf swelling by >3 cm when compared with the asymptomatic leg (measured below the tibial tuberosity)	1
Pitting edema (greater in the symptomatic leg)	1
Collateral superficial veins (nonvaricose)	1
Alternative diagnosis as likely or more likely than that of DVT	−2
Score	
High probability	3 or greater
Moderate probability	1–2
Low probability	0 or less
Modification To compute the modified Wells score, add a point if there is a prior history of documented DVT; using this modified score, DVT is designated as likely or unlikely as follows	
DVT likely	2 or greater
DVT unlikely	1 or less

Data from Refs.[5–8]

Table 5
Wells score for PE

Clinical Feature	Score
Previous PE or DVT	1.5
Heart rate >100 bpm	1.5
Recent surgery or immobilization	1.5
Clinical signs of DVT	3
Alternative diagnosis less likely than PE	3
Hemoptysis	1
Cancer	1
Score	
Low pretest probability	0–1
Intermediate pretest probability	2–6
High pretest probability	≥7

Data from Refs.[5–8]

in patients with contraindications to PE-CT, such as renal dysfunction or severe contrast allergy.

Integrated Diagnostic Approach to the Patient with Suspected Deep Venous Thrombosis

A Wells score for DVT should be computed. If this results in a high pretest probability of DVT, the patient should undergo venous ultrasonography (**Fig. 2**). A positive ultrasound in a patient with a high pretest probability confirms DVT. If a patient with a high pretest probability has a negative ultrasound, a D dimer should be measured, and if this value is greater than 500, a repeat ultrasound should be performed in 1 week. If it is less than or equal to 500, then DVT is ruled out.

For patients with a low pretest probability of DVT, a D dimer should be performed, and if it is negative DVT is ruled out. If D dimer is greater than 500, then a venous ultrasound should be performed, and if negative DVT is ruled out.[15]

Integrated Diagnostic Approach to the Patient with Suspected Pulmonary Embolism

A Wells score for PE should be computed. For patients with a low pretest probability based on Wells and who also fulfill all of the PERC criteria, no further work-up is

Table 6
PE rule-out criteria

Clinical Feature	Score
Age <50 y	1
Initial heart rate <100 bpm	1
Initial oxygen saturation >94% on room air	1
No unilateral leg swelling	1
No hemoptysis	1
No surgery or trauma within 4 wk	1
No history of venous thromboembolism	1
No estrogen use	1
Pretest probability of PE with score 0 is <1%	

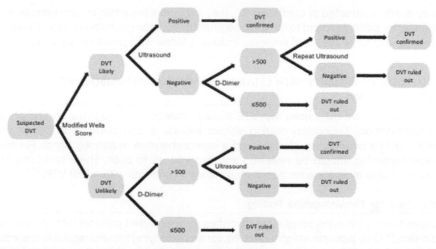

Fig. 2. Diagnostic algorithm for the evaluation of patients with suspected DVT. (*Adapted from* Huisman MV, Klok FA. Diagnostic management of acute deep vein thrombosis and pulmonary embolism. J Thromb Haemost 2013;11(3):418.)

warranted (**Fig. 3**). For patients who have a low-risk Wells score and do not fulfill all of the PERC criteria and those with an intermediate-risk Wells score, a D dimer should be obtained. For this subset of patients, a D dimer less than the age-adjusted normal cutoff rules out PE, and no further imaging should be obtained. If the D dimer is higher than the cutoff, then a PE-CT scan should be performed. Patients who are high risk based on Wells score should proceed directly to CT and a D dimer should not be obtained.[16] Although lower extremity venous ultrasounds are not warranted for all

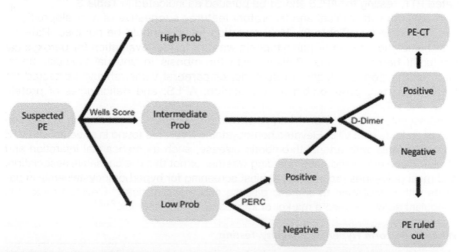

Fig. 3. Diagnostic algorithm for the evaluation of patients with suspected PE. Prob, pretest probability. (*Adapted from* Raja AS, Greenberg JO, Qaseem A, et al. Evaluation of patients with suspected acute pulmonary embolism: best practice advice from the clinical guidelines committee of the American College of Physicians. Ann Intern Med 2015;163(9):704.)

patients with suspected or confirmed PE, they are useful in certain circumstances. For example, for patients found to have subsegmental PE, new guidelines suggest antico-agulation only for a subset of patients, including those with proximal leg DVT.[17]

EVALUATION OF PATIENTS WITH ESTABLISHED VENOUS THROMBOEMBOLI
Routine Evaluation

All patients who are diagnosed with VTE should undergo a thorough history and phys-ical examination. Laboratory testing should include a complete blood count and smear, routine coagulation studies, and a comprehensive metabolic panel. Routine cancer screening should be reviewed and brought up to date. There is no role for more extensive evaluation for occult malignancy in patients with a first VTE.[18]

Indications for Thrombophilia Testing

Routine testing for hypercoagulable disorders in unselected patients with VTE is not indicated.[19] Only patients at increased risk for an underlying hypercoagulable disorder should be tested. Such patients include those with at least one first-degree family member with VTE before age 45, first VTE before age 45, recurrent thrombosis, throm-bosis in unusual vascular beds (eg, portal, hepatic, or cerebral veins), a history of warfarin-induced skin necrosis, or arterial thrombosis.[19]

Evaluation for Thrombophilias

When a decision has been made to test a patient for hypercoagulable disorders, testing should be individualized based on the history, physical examination, and initial laboratory results. Some of the more common tests for inherited thrombophilias include APC/factor V Leiden testing, prothrombin 20210A gene mutation analysis, AT-heparin cofactor assay, and testing for protein C and S deficiency.

In patients with a clinical history that raises suspicion for APLS (eg, a patient with venous and arterial thromboses) or those with an unexplained prolongation of the acti-vated PTT, testing for APLS should be pursued as indicated in **Table 3**.

In patients with clinical and laboratory features suggestive of a myeloprolifera-tive neoplasm (see **Table 2**), JAK2 mutation testing should be pursued. Patients with hemolytic anemia or pancytopenia warrant further evaluation for paroxysmal nocturnal hemoglobinuria. Patients with thrombosis in unusual vascular beds, such as the portal, hepatic, mesenteric, or cerebral veins, should be tested for factor V Leiden; prothrombin gene mutation; APLS; and deficiencies of protein S, C, and AT.

Homocysteine and factor VIII levels should not routinely be checked in the evalua-tion of patients with VTE. Elevated homocysteine levels are found in patients with VTE and in patients with arterial thrombotic disease, such as myocardial infarction and stroke. There are mixed data regarding whether or not this is a causative association, and most guidelines recommend against screening for hyperhomocysteinemia in pa-tients with established thrombotic disease and those at risk.[20] Elevated factor VIII coagulant activity is also a marker of increased thrombotic risk.[21,22]

When to Perform Hypercoagulability Testing

Many of the tests in the hypercoagulable work-up are impacted by acute thrombosis and pharmacologic anticoagulation. If possible, the hypercoagulable testing should be sent at least several weeks after the acute thrombotic event and several weeks after cessation of anticoagulation.

VENOUS THROMBOEMBOLI MANAGEMENT OVERVIEW
Indications for Hospitalization

Many patients with a new diagnosis of VTE can be safely managed as outpatients. Indications for hospitalization include hemodynamic instability, hypoxemia, high risk of bleeding, severe liver or renal disease, thrombocytopenia, concerns for nonadherence, or inadequate home supports.

Advanced Therapies

The management of PE and DVT involves two categories of treatments: advanced therapies that actively break down or remove clot, and anticoagulation. Advanced therapies include embolectomy, most commonly via catheter-based removal of clot, and thrombolysis (ie, the use of agents that break down fibrin clot via activation of plasminogen to its active form plasmin). Although there is growing interest in the use of thrombolysis and embolectomy for prevention of postthrombotic syndrome in patients with symptomatic proximal DVT, advanced therapies are currently not routinely recommended.[17] Patients with acute PE and hypotension should receive systemic thrombolysis unless they have a high bleeding risk. Systemic thrombolysis can also be considered in patients who deteriorate after initiating anticoagulation, provided that they have a low bleeding risk. Catheter-assisted embolectomy should be considered for patients with acute PE and hypotension if they have a high bleeding risk, failed systemic thrombolysis, or if systemic thrombolysis cannot be provided in a reasonable time frame.[17]

Indications for Anticoagulation

Most patients with leg DVT or PE should receive anticoagulation. Patients with DVT/PE who should generally not receive anticoagulation include low-risk patients with subsegmental PE (no involvement of the more proximal pulmonary arteries, no proximal leg DVT, low risk for recurrent DVT), and patients with isolated distal DVT of the leg without severe symptoms or risk factors for extension.[17] Patients with superficial thrombophlebitis and superficial venous thrombosis without concomitant DVT or PE also do not warrant anticoagulation.

ANTICOAGULANTS
Parenteral Anticoagulants

Unfractionated heparin forms a complex with AT that inhibits the activity of factor Xa and thrombin. The low-molecular-weight heparins (LMWH; eg, enoxaparin [Lovenox], dalteparin [Fragmin], and fondaparinux [Arixtra]) are heparin variants that have more predictable pharmacokinetics and more specific anti-Xa action than unfractionated heparin.[23] The parenteral direct thrombin inhibitors include argatroban, bivalirudin (Angiomax), and lepirudin (Refludan).[24] These compounds act by directly binding to and inhibiting thrombin.

Warfarin

Warfarin (Coumadin) is an oral anticoagulant that acts by inhibiting vitamin K oxide reductase, an enzyme essential for the biosynthesis of factors II, VII, IX, and X. Warfarin has a narrow therapeutic window and unpredictable pharmacokinetics that are influenced by diet and other medications.[25] Patients on warfarin therefore must be monitored closely by serial measurement of the international normalized ratio (INR). A major advantage of warfarin is that its effect are reversed with vitamin K, four-factor protein complex concentrate, or fresh frozen plasma.

Direct Oral Anticoagulants

The DOACs include the direct thrombin inhibitor dabigatran (Pradaxa) and the factor Xa inhibitors rivaroxaban (Xarelto), apixaban (Eliquis), and edoxaban (Lixiana) (Table 7). These medications lead to inhibition of rate-limiting steps of coagulation, and inhibition of free and clot-bound factors. Advantages of these medications in comparison with warfarin include lower all-cause mortality (stemming from reduction in fatal intracranial hemorrhages) and less frequent need for monitoring because of more consistent drug effect at a given dose.[26-28] The DOACs all have an onset of action within hours; however, only rivaroxaban and apixaban have been proven in trials to be efficacious without an initial course of parenteral anticoagulation. Patients in the trials that evaluated dabigatran and edoxaban were treated with an initial course of heparin, so these medications are typically started only after at least 5 days of LMWH (see Table 7).

However, there are some important drawbacks to their use. DOACs are more costly than warfarin, cannot easily be reliably monitored, generally lack specific reversal agents, have shorter half-lives leading to greater risk of subtherapeutic levels in the case of missed doses, and some require twice daily dosing. Drug-drug interactions are generally less problematic with DOACs than with warfarin, but medications that induce or inhibit the P-glycoprotein transport system and/or the hepatic cytochrome P-450 CYP3A4 (eg, carbamazepine, rifampin, and ketoconazole) should generally be avoided because they can unpredictably alter DOAC blood levels.

ANTICOAGULANT THERAPY FOR VENOUS THROMBOEMBOLI
Choice of Anticoagulant

There are several important considerations when choosing an anticoagulation regimen and determining the duration of treatment of a patient with VTE. These include the patient's bleeding risk, which is important in weighing risks/benefits of prescribing anticoagulation and in choosing whether or not to prescribe an anticoagulant with an available reversal agent. It is important to consider the patient's medical history, including renal and hepatic dysfunction that may impact the metabolism and/or interfere with monitoring of the chosen anticoagulant.

For most patients, the DOACs are the preferred agents for VTE treatment rather than warfarin.[17,29-33] Patients who are pregnant or who have malignancy-associated VTE should be preferentially prescribed LMWH.[34] DOACs should not be used for patients with prosthetic heart valves because of an increased risk for valve thrombosis.[35] DOACs are renally excreted to variable degrees, so warfarin may be a better choice in patients with renal insufficiency. There are ongoing clinical trials evaluating the efficacy of DOACs for patients with APLS; however, at this point there is not sufficient data to suggest that DOACs are safe in this patient population.[36]

Duration of Anticoagulation

Duration of anticoagulation for VTE should be individualized, taking into consideration the patient's risk of bleeding or recurrent thrombosis. Bleeding risk factors include history of bleed, history of stroke, age, abnormal renal or liver function, thrombocytopenia, hypertension, concomitant antiplatelet therapy, alcohol abuse, frequent falls, and lifestyle factors that lead to a higher risk of bleeding (eg, high-risk jobs or sports activities). The HAS-BLED score can be used to quantitatively assess a patient's bleeding risk.[37]

In general, patients with a first provoked PE or DVT that warrants treatment should receive anticoagulation for 3 months.[17] The most recent CHEST Guidelines do not

Table 7
Direct oral anticoagulants

Characteristic	Dabigatran Etexilate (Pradaxa)	Rivaroxaban (Xarelto)	Apixaban (Eliquis)	Edoxaban (Lixiana)
Initial therapy	LMWH for at least 5 d	15 mg BID for 21 d	10 mg BID for 7 d	LMWH for at least 5 d
Long-term therapy	150 mg BID	20 mg Qday (Consider 15 mg Qday if CrCl 15-50 and high risk of bleeding day 22 onward)	5 mg BID day 8 onward	60 mg Qday (30 mg Qday if CreCl 30-50 mL/min, body weight ≤60 kg or concomitant teatment with potent P-glycoprotein inhibitors)
Extended therapy	150 mg BID	20 mg Qday (Consider 15 mg Qday if CrCl 15-50 and high risk of bleeding day 22 onward)	Dose reduction to 2.5 mg BID after 6 months of anticoagulation	60 mg Qday (30 mg Qday if CreCl 30-50 mL/min, body weight ≤ 60 kg or concomitant teatment with potent P-glycoprotein inhibitors)
Intake with food	Not necessary	Mandatory	Not necessary	Not necessary
Use in renal insufficiency	Contraindicated if CrCl < 30 mL/min	Not recommended if CrCl < 15 mL/min	Not recommended if CrCl < 15 mL/min	Dose adjustments in some cases
Use in the elderly	110 mg BID for patients ≥ 80 y or patients > 75 y with renal impairment or simultaneous treatment with a strong P-glycoprotein inhibitor			
Antidote	Idarucizumab	Under development	Under development	Under development

Abbreviation: CrCl, creatinine clearance.

support extending the duration of anticoagulation beyond 3 months for provoked VTE.[17] Patients with unprovoked PE or DVT should receive anticoagulation for 3 months if they have a high bleeding risk and indefinitely if their bleeding risk is lower.[17] In some patients with unprovoked DVT and high bleeding risk, it is helpful to risk stratify with a repeat ultrasound and/or D dimer before stopping anticoagulation at 3 months, and to consider continuing anticoagulation in patients with evidence of significant persistent clot. There are no consensus guidelines regarding use of repeat D dimer or ultrasound in this manner.[38] Patients with unprovoked proximal DVT or PE who stop anticoagulation therapy should be considered for aspirin monotherapy.[17]

Direct Oral Anticoagulant Patient Monitoring

Before starting a DOAC, a baseline basic metabolic panel, liver functional tests, complete blood count, INR, and PTT should be measured. DOACs variably affect the PTT and INR but these parameters cannot be relied on to monitor drug effect. Patients on DOACs should have clinic visits at least every 6 months.[39] At these visits, they should have a blood pressure and creatinine measurement. Their adherence should be assessed, and they should be counseled on the importance of not missing doses of DOAC. They should be assessed for bleeding risks and possible new interacting medications.

Management of Direct Oral Anticoagulant Bleeding Complications

The DOACs do not all have specific reversal agents. Although bleeding risks are low, there is a risk of severe bleeding.[32] General management of severe DOAC-associated bleeding includes cessation of the DOAC, oral activated charcoal if the last DOAC dose was within the previous few hours, anatomic management of the hemorrhage (eg, surgical or endoscopic intervention), and administration of antifibrinolytic agents (eg, tranexamic acid [Cyklokapron] or aminocaproic acid [Amicar]). Hemodialysis should be considered in patients on dabigatran; this is not useful for the factor Xa inhibitors because they are not dialyzable. Patients on dabigatran with major bleeding can be given idarucizumab (Praxbind), a specific antidote.[40] Protein complex concentrate should be considered in patients with major bleeding on factor Xa inhibitors. Andexanet alfa and ciraparantag are other DOAC antidotes currently in the pipeline but not yet approved by the Food and Drug Administration for clinical use.[41,42]

VENOUS THROMBOEMBOLI PROPHYLAXIS
Primary Prophylaxis

Primary prophylaxis for VTE is indicated for hospitalized patients. Patients who are chronically immobilized do not warrant prophylactic pharmacologic anticoagulation beyond their first 3 months of immobility.[43] Pharmacologic VTE prophylaxis should be considered for patients at above average VTE risk on long plane, train, or car trips, but is not indicated for patients at average risk.[44]

Secondary Venous Thromboemboli Prophylaxis Other Than Chronic Anticoagulation

Patients who are diagnosed with VTE should be counseled regarding lifestyle modifications that decrease their risk of VTE recurrence, including weight loss, increased exercise, and smoking cessation. Patients should be advised of their increased clotting risk with estrogen therapy and with pregnancy.

SUMMARY

Venous thromboembolic disease is an important cause of morbidity and mortality. Key recent practice shifts include the refinement of evidence-based algorithms for VTE diagnosis and the emergence of the DOACs as first-line therapies. It is likely that going forward use of DOACs will expand even further as more data emerge regarding their safety in specialized populations (eg, malignancy, pregnancy) and as additional DOAC reversal agents become available.

REFERENCES

1. Heit JA. The epidemiology of venous thromboembolism in the community. Arterioscler Thromb Vasc Biol 2008;28(3):370–2.
2. Goldhaber SZ. Venous thromboembolism: epidemiology and magnitude of the problem. Best Pract Res Clin Haematol 2012;25(3):235–42.
3. Gavish I, Brenner B. Air travel and the risk of thromboembolism. Intern Emerg Med 2011;6(2):113–6.
4. Stein PD, Beemath A, Matta F, et al. Clinical characteristics of patients with acute pulmonary embolism: data from PIOPED II. Am J Med 2007;120(10):871–9.
5. Wells PS, Anderson DR, Rodger M, et al. Derivation of a simple clinical model to categorize patients probability of pulmonary embolism: increasing the models utility with the SimpliRED D-dimer. Thromb Haemost 2000;83(3):416–20.
6. Gibson NS, Sohne M, Kruip MJ, et al. Further validation and simplification of the Wells clinical decision rule in pulmonary embolism. Thromb Haemost 2008;99(1): 229–34.
7. Wells PS, Anderson DR, Bormanis J, et al. Value of assessment of pretest probability of deep-vein thrombosis in clinical management. Lancet 1997;350(9094): 1795–8.
8. Wells PS, Anderson DR, Rodger M, et al. Evaluation of D-dimer in the diagnosis of suspected deep-vein thrombosis. N Engl J Med 2003;349(13):1227–35.
9. Kline JA, Webb WB, Jones AE, et al. Impact of a rapid rule-out protocol for pulmonary embolism on the rate of screening, missed cases, and pulmonary vascular imaging in an urban US emergency department. Ann Emerg Med 2004;44(5):490–502.
10. Kline JA, Courtney DM, Kabrhel C, et al. Prospective multicenter evaluation of the pulmonary embolism rule-out criteria. J Thromb Haemost 2008;6(5):772–80.
11. Kline JA, Peterson CE, Steuerwald MT. Prospective evaluation of real-time use of the pulmonary embolism rule-out criteria in an academic emergency department. Acad Emerg Med 2010;17(9):1016–9.
12. Singh B, Mommer SK, Erwin PJ, et al. Pulmonary embolism rule-out criteria (PERC) in pulmonary embolism–revisited: a systematic review and meta-analysis. Emerg Med J 2013;30(9):701–6.
13. Righini M, Van Es J, Exter Den PL, et al. Age-adjusted D-dimer cutoff levels to rule out pulmonary embolism: the ADJUST-PE study. JAMA 2014;311(11):1117–24.
14. Schouten HJ, Geersing GJ, Koek HL, et al. Diagnostic accuracy of conventional or age adjusted D-dimer cut-off values in older patients with suspected venous thromboembolism: systematic review and meta-analysis. BMJ 2013;346:f2492.
15. Huisman MV, Klok FA. Diagnostic management of acute deep vein thrombosis and pulmonary embolism. J Thromb Haemost 2013;11(3):412–22.
16. Raja AS, Greenberg JO, Qaseem A, et al. Evaluation of patients with suspected acute pulmonary embolism: best practice advice from the clinical guidelines

Committee of the American College of Physicians. Ann Intern Med 2015;163(9): 701–11.

17. Kearon C, Akl EA, Ornelas J, et al. Antithrombotic Therapy for VTE Disease: CHEST Guideline and Expert Panel Report. Chest 2016;149(2):315–52.

18. Carrier M, Lazo-Langner A, Shivakumar S, et al. Screening for occult cancer in unprovoked venous thromboembolism. N Engl J Med 2015;373(8):697–704.

19. Baglin T, Gray E, Greaves M, et al. Clinical guidelines for testing for heritable thrombophilia. Br J Haematol 2010;149(2):209–20.

20. U.S. Preventive Services Task Force. Using nontraditional risk factors in coronary heart disease risk assessment: U.S. Preventive Services Task Force recommendation statement. Ann Intern Med 2009;151(7):474–82.

21. Tsai AW, Cushman M, Rosamond WD, et al. Coagulation factors, inflammation markers, and venous thromboembolism: the longitudinal investigation of thromboembolism etiology (LITE). Am J Med 2002;113(8):636–42.

22. Koster T, Vandenbroucke JP, Briët E, et al. Role of clotting factor VIII in effect of von Willebrand factor on occurrence of deep-vein thrombosis. Lancet 1995; 345(8943):152–5.

23. Hirsh J, Bauer KA, Donati MB, et al. Parenteral anticoagulants: American College of Chest Physicians Evidence-Based Clinical Practice Guidelines (8th Edition). Chest 2008;133(6 Suppl):141S–59S.

24. Di Nisio M, Middeldorp S, Buller HR. Direct thrombin inhibitors. N Engl J Med 2005;353(10):1028–40.

25. Ansell J, Hirsh J, Hylek E, et al. Pharmacology and management of the vitamin K antagonists: American College of Chest Physicians Evidence-Based Clinical Practice Guidelines (8th Edition). Chest 2008;133(6 Suppl):160S–98S.

26. Connolly SJ, Ezekowitz MD, Yusuf S, et al. Dabigatran versus warfarin in patients with atrial fibrillation. N Engl J Med 2009;361(12):1139–51.

27. Patel MR, Mahaffey KW, Garg J, et al. Rivaroxaban versus warfarin in nonvalvular atrial fibrillation. N Engl J Med 2011;365(10):883–91.

28. Granger CB, Alexander JH, McMurray JJV, et al. Apixaban versus warfarin in patients with atrial fibrillation. N Engl J Med 2011;365(11):981–92.

29. EINSTEIN Investigators, Bauersachs R, Berkowitz SD, et al. Oral rivaroxaban for symptomatic venous thromboembolism. N Engl J Med 2010;363(26):2499–510.

30. Agnelli G, Buller HR, Cohen A, et al. Oral apixaban for the treatment of acute venous thromboembolism. N Engl J Med 2013;369(9):799–808.

31. EINSTEIN–PE Investigators, Buller HR, Prins MH, et al. Oral rivaroxaban for the treatment of symptomatic pulmonary embolism. N Engl J Med 2012;366(14): 1287–97.

32. Chai-Adisaksopha C, Hillis C, Isayama T, et al. Mortality outcomes in patients receiving direct oral anticoagulants: a systematic review and meta-analysis of randomized controlled trials. J Thromb Haemost 2015;13(11):2012–20.

33. Schulman S, Kearon C, Kakkar AK, et al. Dabigatran versus warfarin in the treatment of acute venous thromboembolism. N Engl J Med 2009;361(24):2342–52.

34. Lee AYY, Levine MN, Baker RI, et al. Low-molecular-weight heparin versus a Coumadin for the prevention of recurrent venous thromboembolism in patients with cancer. N Engl J Med 2003;349(2):146–53.

35. Eikelboom JW, Brueckmann M, van de Werf F. Dabigatran versus warfarin in patients with mechanical heart valves: reply. J Thromb Haemost 2014;12(3):426.

36. Chighizola CB, Moia M, Meroni PL. New oral anticoagulants in thrombotic antiphospholipid syndrome. Lupus 2014;23(12):1279–82.

37. Lip GYH. Implications of the CHA(2)DS(2)-VASc and HAS-BLED Scores for thromboprophylaxis in atrial fibrillation. Am J Med 2011;124(2):111–4.
38. Stephenson EJP, Liem TK. Duplex imaging of residual venous obstruction to guide duration of therapy for lower extremity deep venous thrombosis. J Vasc Surg Venous Lymphat Disord 2015;3(3):326–32.
39. Gladstone DJ, Geerts WH, Douketis J, et al. How to monitor patients receiving direct oral anticoagulants for stroke prevention in atrial fibrillation: a practice tool endorsed by thrombosis Canada, the Canadian Stroke Consortium, the Canadian Cardiovascular Pharmacists Network, and the Canadian Cardiovascular Society. Ann Intern Med 2015;163(5):382–5.
40. Pollack CV, Reilly PA, Eikelboom J, et al. Idarucizumab for dabigatran reversal. N Engl J Med 2015;373(6):511–20.
41. Siegal DM, Curnutte JT, Connolly SJ, et al. Andexanet Alfa for the reversal of factor Xa inhibitor activity. N Engl J Med 2015;373(25):2413–24.
42. Ansell JE, Bakhru SH, Laulicht BE, et al. Use of PER977 to reverse the anticoagulant effect of edoxaban. N Engl J Med 2014;371(22):2141–2.
43. Gatt ME, Paltiel O, Bursztyn M. Is prolonged immobilization a risk factor for symptomatic venous thromboembolism in elderly bedridden patients? Results of a historical-cohort study. Thromb Haemost 2004;91(3):538–43.
44. Belcaro G, Cesarone MR, Nicolaides AN, et al. Prevention of venous thrombosis with elastic stockings during long-haul flights: the LONFLIT 5 JAP study. Clin Appl Thromb Hemost 2003;9(3):197–201.

Bleeding Diatheses
Approach to the Patient Who Bleeds or Has Abnormal Coagulation

Marcia Paddock, MD, PhD*, John Chapin, MD

KEYWORDS

- Bleeding disorders • Coagulation • von Willebrand disease • Hemophilia
- Platelet defects

KEY POINTS

- Abnormal bleeding is commonly first encountered in the primary care office and may be due to medication or an underlying bleeding disorder.
- A thorough bleeding history and interpretation of basic laboratory tests, such as complete blood count, prothrombin time, and activated partial thromboplastin time can help elucidate the cause of bleeding.
- Common medications, such as aspirin, vitamin K antagonists (warfarin), or oral anticoagulants, can cause bleeding and can cause abnormal coagulation studies.
- Inherited bleeding conditions, including von Willebrand disease, hemophilia, or platelet disorders, often can be diagnosed in the primary care setting, although diagnosis of a bleeding disorder should prompt referral to a hematologist.

ESTABLISHING A DIAGNOSIS

Understanding bleeding diatheses requires a basic understanding of normal hemostasis and coagulation. Under normal conditions, the free flow of blood is maintained within an intact vascular system by multiple safeguards, including the endothelial lining, which produces anticoagulant factors, such as nitric oxide and prostacyclin, and obscures procoagulant factors, such as tissue factor (TF).[1] However, when there is a hemostatic challenge, as after injury, a complex cascade of coagulation is initiated to prevent excessive blood loss. Various alterations to this system, whether by genetic mutation or taking medication, may prevent normal hemostasis and is discussed in this article.

Department of Medicine, Division of Hematology and Medical Oncology, Weill Cornell Medicine and New York Presbyterian Hospital, 520 East 70th Street, Starr Pavilion, 3rd Floor, New York, NY 10065, USA
* Corresponding author.
E-mail address: mnp9005@nyp.org

Prim Care Clin Office Pract 43 (2016) 637–650
http://dx.doi.org/10.1016/j.pop.2016.07.009   primarycare.theclinics.com

Overview of Hemostasis and Coagulation Studies

Primary hemostasis consists initially of platelet adhesion to TF, collagen, von Wille-brand factor (vWF), and fibronectin on the subendothelial matrix that becomes exposed during injury or endothelial damage. After this initial contact, the platelets become activated resulting in increased expression of surface proteins and release of granules that contain factors to further enhance coagulation. The platelets then aggregate with each other through binding of fibrinogen with glycoprotein IIb-IIIa to form a platelet plug.[2] Secondary hemostasis refers to the role of the clotting cascade in generating thrombin, which also activates fibrinogen to fibrin and further supports the initial platelet plug. Finally, the newly formed fibrin mesh is cross-linked by factor XIIIa to form a thrombus.

The clotting cascade is divided into the extrinsic, intrinsic, and common pathways (**Fig. 1**). The extrinsic pathway (also known as the TF pathway) is initiated by the binding of TF by factor VII, which generates the prothrombinase complex, composed of the common pathway components factor Xa, factor Va, calcium, and phospholipids. The prothrombinase complex activates prothrombin to thrombin, which in turn converts fibrinogen to fibrin, as discussed previously. The extrinsic pathway is thought to be the primary method of activating the clotting cascade in vivo and is critical for normal he-mostasis.[3] This pathway is measured through the prothrombin time (PT) test (**Table 1**).

The intrinsic pathway (so named because in a test tube it does not require the addi-tion of TF to initiate this pathway) is composed of factors XII, XI, IX, and VIII, which generate the prothrombinase complex, as described previously. The intrinsic pathway is initiated in vitro by interaction with a negatively charged surface, such as silica or kaolin, and is measured through the activated partial thromboplastin time (aPTT). In vivo, this process is initiated by the extrinsic pathway, but may also be activated by artificial surfaces and chains of inorganic polyphosphates released from platelet granules on activation.[4]

Thrombin is the key point in the clotting cascade where the pathways converge, and it plays an important role in coagulation, not just through activating fibrinogen and platelets but is also a primary site of regulation of coagulation. Thrombin in part serves as its own regulator through a negative feedback loop initiated by activating protein C, protein S, and antithrombin, which are natural anticoagulants and serve as inhibitors of the clotting cascade (see **Fig. 1**).

Taking a Bleeding History and Physical Examination

When a patient presents for an evaluation of abnormal bleeding, a thorough history is an essential first step. The physician must assess whether the amount of bleeding the pa-tient experiences is truly abnormal. This can be difficult, and formalized approaches have been developed, including bleeding tools. However, multiple studies have shown that it can be difficult to assess severity of bleeding by questionnaire. Several tools, such as the Vincenza bleeding score, ISTH-BAT (International Society on Thrombosis and Hemostasis Bleeding Assessment Tool), or the MCMDM (Condensed Molecular and Clinical Markers for the Diagnosis and Management of Type 1 VWD Bleeding Ques-tionnaire) have been developed to help take an accurate and reproducible bleeding his-tory; however, they have been robustly validated only in von Willebrand disease (vWD).[5–7] In a study of 500 healthy individuals conducted by a trained physician or nurse practitioner, nearly three-quarters of respondents reported bleeding symptoms, including 25% of respondents reporting epistaxis, 18% reporting easy bruising, and 47% of women reporting heavy menses.[8] In children, the frequency of reporting bleeding symptoms may be even higher.[9]

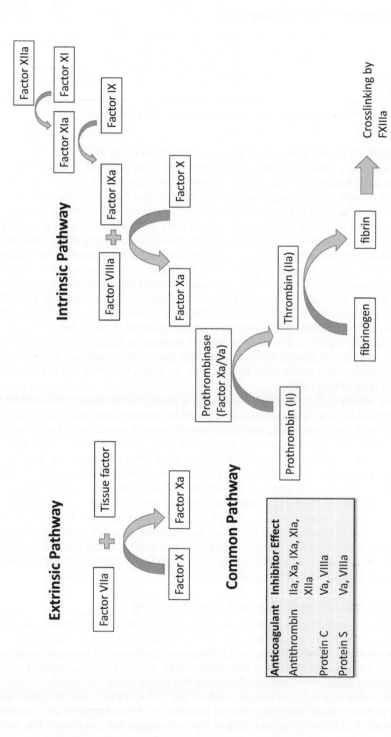

Fig. 1. Pathways of the clotting cascade.

Table 1	
Prolonged coagulation tests and diagnosis	
Prolonged PT	Factor VII deficiency, warfarin use, vitamin K deficiency, lupus anticoagulant
Prolonged aPTT	Factor deficiency (Factors VIII, IX, XI, XII), heparin anticoagulation, argatroban anticoagulation, lupus anticoagulant
Prolonged PT and aPTT	Factor deficiency (Factors II, V, X, fibrinogen), vitamin K deficiency

Abbreviations: aPTT, activated partial thromboplastin time; PT, prothrombin time.

When taking a bleeding history, specific questions are often more useful than open-ended ones, and a complete history starts with birth. The onset of abnormal bleeding is important, as it will often help distinguish between a congenital disorder and an acquired one, which may correlate with a new medication or procedure. Questions to help determine the onset of a bleeding disorder include whether the patient had umbilical stump bleeding, bleeding with circumcision, history of childhood traumas, epistaxis, and a complete menstrual and obstetric history. In addition, asking about prior hemostatic challenges, including previous surgeries and dental procedures, will assist in determining if a patient has a true bleeding diathesis. Subjective questions such as "Are your periods heavy?" should be exchanged for more objective ones to try to quantify the bleeding such as "How many pads or tampons do you saturate in a day?" or "Have you ever required a blood transfusion for your bleeding? If so, how many units?"

A thorough medication history including any supplements the patient takes and a complete family history are also important in assessing abnormal bleeding. Many common medications disrupt platelet function or the clotting cascade, especially cardiac medications and some over-the-counter analgesics, which will be discussed separately later in this article.

As many bleeding diatheses are hereditary, a strong family history of bleeding is a convincing reason to initiate a workup for a possible bleeding disorder. In general, a history of mucocutaneous bleeding, such as gingival bleeding, nosebleeds, heavy menses, or bleeding after childbirth, are more suggestive of a platelet problem (thrombocytopenia, dysfunctional platelets, or vWD). Bleeding into joints or deep tissues is more suggestive of a coagulation factor deficiency (including congenital or acquired hemophilia).

A physical examination also can provide additional information about a bleeding diathesis. Significant findings include bruises on arms or legs, where there may have been trauma, versus on the trunk or face, where trauma is less likely to go unnoticed. Petechiae in dependent areas, such as the lower legs and also on the palate, suggest a platelet disorder. Telangiectasias in the mouth and nose could be associated with hemorrhagic hereditary telangiectasia and the murmur of aortic stenosis could indicate acquired vWD or Heyde syndrome.

Initial Laboratory Testing to Work up Excessive Bleeding

The first steps to initiating a laboratory evaluation of abnormal bleeding include a complete blood count with a platelet count, review of a peripheral blood smear, and coagulation studies starting with PT and aPTT. These tests will identify many of the patients with abnormal bleeding, including thrombocytopenia (discussed elsewhere) and the most common factor deficiencies. Review of the blood smear is required to rule out pseudothrombocytopenia, an artifact in which the EDTA in the collection tube causes platelets to clump such that they are not counted by the automated cell counter.[10] Finding even 1 platelet clump invalidates the automated cell count and the platelet count should be repeated in a citrate tube or a blood smear made directly at the bedside. If these initial tests are normal, the next steps include platelet studies, such as PFA-100, platelet aggregometry, and von Willebrand factor studies with multimer analysis. These tests will detect vWD, medications that affect platelet function, or intrinsic platelet defects. Abnormal findings on these tests in the setting of bleeding should prompt discussions with a coagulation specialist.

Interpretation of Coagulation Studies

Prothrombin time and international normalized ratio

PT and international normalized ratio (INR) are used to determine abnormalities in the extrinsic or TF pathway, as well as the common pathway (factors I, II, V, and X). It is performed by adding calcium, phospholipid, and TF to citrated plasma. The INR was developed to standardize the PT test, which otherwise was variable between laboratories due to variations in TF preparations. It should be noted that the INR is a way of monitoring levels of vitamin K antagonists, such as warfarin.[11] It is not a validated tool to assess bleeding risk in other contexts. For example, in liver failure, INR increases due to inability to synthesize clotting factors II, VII, IX, and X in the liver; however, these patients have increased clotting risk due to lack of natural anticoagulants, which are also synthesized in the liver and their bleeding risk is not reliably predicted by INR.[12] Rarely in the outpatient setting will a patient be so malnourished as to have a nutritional vitamin K deficiency, but this should also be considered when testing reveals a prolonged PT/INR.

Activated partial thromboplastin time

aPTT measures the intrinsic and common pathways of coagulation, and is also used to monitor the therapeutic effect of certain anticoagulants, such as heparin and argatroban. It is performed by adding calcium and a partial activated thromboplastin reagent to plasma collected with citrate and measuring the time to clot formation. An elevated aPTT can be seen in deficiencies of factor VIII, IX, XI, or other components of the contact pathway. When a blood sample is contaminated with heparin, or a lupus anticoagulant is present, the aPTT will be prolonged (see **Table 1**).

A shortened PT or aPTT may be seen in times of critical illness due to an excess of TF (PT) or factor VIII (aPTT) but the significance of this is not clear with respect to coagulation risk.

Mixing studies

An elevated PT or aPTT may suggest an abnormality of the clotting cascade and should be followed up with a mixing study. A mixing study is performed by adding pooled normal plasma to the patient's plasma in a 1:1 ratio and measuring the PT or aPTT immediately, and followed by incubation of 60 to 120 minutes at 37°C. If the aPTT corrects immediately on mixing and remains corrected in the incubated sample, this suggests a deficiency of a factor that is replaced by the normal plasma. An acquired inhibitor to FVIII exhibits a time-dependent binding, and thus the incubated aPTT will become prolonged only after incubation. If the clotting time does not correct at either time point, it is most consistent with an antiphospholipid antibody, which causes thrombosis, not bleeding (**Table 2**).

The PT and aPTT are both dependent on functional fibrinogen, as it is required to form a clot in the assay. In patients with severe liver disease causing dysfunctional fibrinogen, both tests may be prolonged. An "indeterminate" test may result if there is not enough fibrinogen to form a clot with sufficient viscosity or optical density to trigger the automated analyzer.

Table 2 Interpretation of 1:1 mixing study		
Immediate Correction?	**Correction After Incubation?**	**Diagnosis**
Yes	Yes	Factor deficiency
No	No	Lupus anticoagulant
Yes	No	Factor inhibitor (eg, acquired hemophilia A)

Effects of Medications on Coagulation

Warfarin is a vitamin K antagonist commonly used as an anticoagulant. Vitamin K is an essential cofactor for the activation of factors II, VII, IX, X, protein C, and protein S and therapeutic levels of warfarin are maintained by following the PT/INR. The oral direct Xa inhibitors, such as apixaban, rivaroxaban, and edoxaban, also can cause a prolongation of the PT or aPTT, but not in predictable ways, thus rendering these tests unsuitable for monitoring the levels of the drugs. Other tests that rely on clotting times, such as screening tests for lupus anticoagulant, cannot always be reliably performed when a patient is on warfarin or other anticoagulation.

Platelet Studies

Platelet functional assays, such as the PFA-100 and platelet aggregometry, measure qualitative platelet defects. The PFA-100 test was designed to replace the bleeding time test and measures how long a sample of whole blood takes to clot when passed through a special chamber in which platelets are activated by either collagen-epinephrine or collagen-ADP.[13] Aspirin and nonsteroidal anti-inflammatory drugs (NSAIDs) may cause a prolongation of the collagen-epinephrine aggregation time and clopidogrel may prolong aggregation time in both columns. Both chambers also will take longer to aggregate in the setting of uremic platelet dysfunction, vWD, or liver disease. If more specific testing is required, complete platelet aggregometry can be performed. Complete aggregometry includes a panel of platelet agonists, including ADP, epinephrine, collagen, a thromboxane A2 mimetic, arachidonic acid, thrombin receptor activating peptide, and ristocetin.[14] By correlating which platelet agonists are able to induce aggregation and which do not, specific defects in platelet function can be determined.

Several medications that patients take may have an effect on these assays. Abnormal test results will be found in the setting of antiplatelet medications, such as clopidogrel or ticagrelor, over-the-counter medications, such as aspirin, NSAIDs, guaifenesin, some herbal supplements such as fish oil, or certain antidepressants, all of which can affect platelet function and hemostasis.

SPECIFIC BLEEDING DIAGNOSES AND TREATMENT
von Willebrand Disease

vWD is the most common congenital bleeding disorder, with an estimated prevalence of up to 1%, although the bleeding phenotype is variable. In assessing vWD, several tests are commonly ordered that assay several aspects of vWF, including the following:

- Antigen level (vWF:Ag): a quantitative measure of the protein without information on its function
- Activity (vWF:RCo): a functional assay that measures platelet aggregation after addition of the activator ristocetin

- vWF:RCo/vWF:Ag ratio: the ratio between antigen and activity levels, which can help distinguish type I from type II vWD
- Factor VIII activity: vWF is required to maintain FVIII in circulation
- vWF multimers: vWF circulates as a large multimer, and electrophoresis for multimer size also helps to distinguish subtypes of vWD.

vWD is classified into 3 main types (**Table 3**). Type I is a quantitative deficiency of vWF and can be mild, moderate, or severe, depending on the degree of the protein deficiency. In von Willebrand assays, this will result in both low von Willebrand antigen and activity, maintaining a preserved vWF:RCo/vWF:Ag ratio.

Type II vWD is a qualitative deficiency of vWF activity characterized by a decreased ratio of vWF:RCo/vWF:Ag (often <0.7). There are multiple subtypes of type II vWD, including IIA, IIB, IIM, and IIN, each characterized by a different defect:

- vWD IIA is the most common subtype and is caused by a deficiency of high molecular weight (HMW) multimers of vWF, which reduces the efficiency of binding to platelets.
- vWD IIB is a gain-of-function mutation that causes increased binding to platelet glycoprotein Ib.[15] This binding occurs even in settings without hemostatic challenge leading to a consumption of platelets and the larger vWF multimers. As such, treatment of bleeding with DDAVP (desmopressin) is relatively contraindicated due to the risk of worsening bleeding by increasing the consumption of platelets.
- vWD IIM is a defect in the ability of vWF to bind platelets (loss of function mutation causing decreased binding to platelet glycoprotein 1b). Although there are normal levels of the vWF protein and normal HMW multimers, there is a decrease

Table 3
Laboratory characteristics of von Willebrand's disease by subtype

vWD Subtype	aPTT	vWF:Ag	vWF:RCo	VIII:C	RCo:Ag Ratio	Multimers
I – Reduced vWF protein expression	Normal-to-prolonged	Reduced	Reduced	Normal-to-reduced	Normal	Normal
IIA – Deficiency of HMW multimers	Normal-to-prolonged	Mildly reduced	Reduced	Normal-to-reduced	Reduced	Reduced HMW
IIB – Increased platelet binding and consumption of HMW multimers	Normal-to-prolonged	Mildly reduced	Reduced	Normal-to-reduced	Reduced	Variable loss of HMW
IIM – Defect in interactions with platelets	Normal-to-prolonged	Mildly reduced	Reduced	Normal-to-reduced	Reduced	Normal
IIN – Defective binding and stabilization of FVIII	Prolonged	Normal	Normal	Reduced	Normal	Normal
III – Absent vWF protein	Prolonged	Absent	Absent	Reduced	Not applicable	Absent

Abbreviations: aPTT, activated partial thromboplastin time; HMW, high molecular weight; PT, prothrombin time; vWD, von Willebrand disease; vWF, von Willebrand factor; vWF:Ag, a quantitative measure of the protein without information on its function; vWF:RCo, a functional assay that measures platelet aggregation after addition of the activator ristocetin.

in vWF activity as measured by platelet aggregation in response to activation with ristocetin.

- vWD IIN (Normandy) subtype is caused by mutations that decrease the ability of vWF to bind and stabilize FVIII, causing a prolonged aPTT and low FVIII levels on testing. Because of the decreased FVIII levels, type IIN vWD can be confused with hemophilia A on preliminary testing and care must be taken to establish the correct diagnosis.

Type III vWD is an absence of von Willebrand factor and is characterized by an absent vWF:Ag. This is extremely rare and is often associated with a severe bleeding phenotype.

Minor bleeding in the setting of vWD is often treated with DDAVP, which can be effective in patients with type I and some patients with type II vWD. DDAVP causes the release of vWF stores in endothelial cells and platelets and can be sufficient to stop a minor bleed. However, the benefit of DDAVP is short-lived, as the store of pre-made vWF is rapidly depleted after 2 to 3 doses, resulting in tachyphylaxis. Any bleeding sufficient to cause a hemoglobin drop requires vWF replacement. If a patient has vWD, it is recommended they see a hematologist to test the response to DDAVP in a controlled setting and develop an effective bleeding plan for emergencies.

vWD is usually congenital, but also can be acquired. Acquired vWD is commonly seen in the setting of severe aortic stenosis, which produces shear forces that degrade the largest multimers. Loss of HMW vWF multimers is almost always seen in patients with left ventricular assist devices, although interestingly rates of significant bleeding are only approximately 30% and do not seem to directly correlate with vWF levels.[16] One can also acquire vWD secondary to thrombocytosis greater than 1,000,000 platelets, which may be seen in essential thrombocythemia or polycythemia vera due to consumption of vWF on platelet surfaces.[17]

Hemophilia A and B

Hemophilia A is a deficiency of FVIII that is present in 1 in 5,000 to 10,000 male births. Hemophilia demonstrates sex-linked recessive inheritance, which means it is almost exclusively seen in men. Women sometimes can be symptomatic carriers. Hemophilia B is a deficiency of factor IX seen in approximately 1 in 30,000 male births. Clinically, hemophilia B can look very similar to hemophilia A and specific factor activity assay testing is required to distinguish them. In approximately 30% of cases of hemophilia, there is no family history of hemophilia.

Hemophilia can be mild (6%–30% of the normal factor level), moderate (1%–5%), or severe (<1%). Patients with hemophilia can present with ecchymoses (spontaneous bruising without preceding trauma) and bleeding into joints or soft tissues. In severe hemophilia, spontaneous bleeding usually manifests in the first year of life, whereas in moderate or mild hemophilia, presentation can be variable. As hemophilia is caused by a defect in the intrinsic pathway, these patients have a prolonged aPTT, which should prompt measurement of FVIII and/or FIX levels. Patients with severe hemophilia require lifelong prophylactic factor replacement to prevent disabling joint disease from recurrent hemarthrosis. However, patients with moderate disease may still have severe bleeding in response to relatively minor trauma and require factor replacement after injuries or scheduled procedures.

Acquired Hemophilia

Hemophilia also can be acquired through the development of autoantibodies to endogenous FVIII.[18] In contrast to congenital hemophilia, acquired hemophilia is more likely to present with mucocutaneous bleeding or extensive ecchymoses, rather than deep tissue bleeds. Acquired hemophilia is most common in older patients, in whom the development of these autoantibodies is idiopathic, but it can also affect younger individuals in whom it may be associated with pregnancy, autoimmune disease, or malignancies. The diagnosis is often made in the setting of an acute bleed, which should be managed aggressively both with local control of bleeding and use of bypassing agents, such as prothrombin complex concentrates like Factor Eight Inhibitor Bypassing Activity (FEIBA), recombinant factor VIIa, or porcine FVIII. Efforts should also be undertaken to eradicate the autoantibody with agents such as rituximab or cyclophosphamide in idiopathic cases, and treatment of any underlying condition should be initiated.

Factor VIII Inhibitors

Patients with congenital hemophilia who require factor replacement risk the development of antibodies to the exogenous FVIII. Development of inhibitors to FIX is much less common than FVIII. Any patient who has had factor replacement and has worsening bleeding or unexplained elevation in the aPTT should be tested for FVIII inhibitors. In a mixing study, FVIII inhibitors classically have immediate correction and prolonged aPTT in the incubated sample, as previously described. The FVIII inhibitor is quantified by performing serial dilutions with the patient's serum until the inhibitor is reduced to 50% activity and the number of dilutions is reported as Bethesda Units (BU). A stronger inhibitor will have higher BU, indicating it can be diluted more times before its efficacy is reduced. An inhibitor titer greater than 5 BU is unlikely to be overcome with factor replacement alone and may require bypass agents to stop bleeding. The development of inhibitors is most common in the pediatric population, with severe hemophilia requiring prophylactic factor replacement (up to 25%–30%). Although most cases will occur within the first 50 exposures, 3% to 13% of cases are in patients with moderate and mild hemophilia A.[19] Prompt diagnosis is critical and physicians should maintain a high index of suspicion in a patient with mild or moderate hemophilia receiving factor replacement in the setting of surgery or trauma.

Factor XI Deficiency

Factor XI deficiency is seen primarily in Ashkenazi Jewish populations, in which up to 1 in 10 individuals may carry a mutation, although the incidence of a carrier state for this autosomal recessive disorder in the general population is closer to 1 in 100.[20] In contrast to hemophilia A and B, the level of FXI does not accurately predict the bleeding phenotype, as different mutations may have different phenotypes ranging from asymptomatic to severe. Bleeding risk in these patients is best assessed by taking a thorough bleeding history and then factor replacement (eg, fresh frozen plasma) can be used if needed.

Other Factor Deficiencies

Other factor deficiencies, including II, V, VII, X, and XIII, are very rare, occurring in 0.5 to 2 per 1,000,000 individuals and are outlined in **Table 4**. Although one may have an FXII deficiency, it is not associated with a bleeding phenotype, although it may prolong the aPTT. Factors VII, X, and XIII have concentrates available, but in some locations, they may not be readily available during an acute bleed. In the absence of specific factor concentrate, prothrombin complex concentrate (PCC), cryoprecipitate, or fresh frozen plasma (FFP) can be used to replace relevant factors. PCC comes in 3-factor (II, IX, and X) and 4-factor (II, VII, IX, and X) varieties. Cryoprecipitate contains fibrinogen, vWF, FVIII, and FXIII. FFP contains all the clotting factors and is readily available in most clinical settings, although it contains much lower concentrations of factor than

Table 4
Rare factor deficiencies

Factor Deficiency	Laboratory Abnormality	Treatment for Acute Bleeding	Comments
II	PT and aPTT prolonged	PCC or FFP	
V	PT and aPTT prolonged	FFP	May also be treated with platelet transfusions as platelets contain factor V
VII	Isolated PT prolonged	Recombinant Factor VIIa or 4 factor PCC	Phenotype may not correlate with factor level
X	PT and aPTT prolonged	Factor X concentrate or PCC	May be congenital or acquired in amyloidosis
XIII	Normal PT and aPTT	Factor XIII concentrate, cryoprecipitate, or FFP	Routine prophylaxis recommended for severe patients
Afibrinogenemia/ dysfibrinogenemia	PT and aPTT prolonged, thrombin time prolonged	Fibrinogen concentrate or cryoprecipitate	Replacement may be required to maintain pregnancy

Abbreviations: aPTT, activated partial thromboplastin time; FFP, fresh frozen plasma; PCC, prothrombin complex concentrate; PT, prothrombin time.

in concentrates and a larger volume is needed to be given to control bleeding. Prophylaxis can be very useful in afibrinogenemias and XIII deficiency.

PLATELET DISORDERS

Thrombocytopenia can cause bleeding and has many causes (eg, immune thrombocytopenic purpura, medication) discussed elsewhere. Platelet dysfunction in patients with normal platelet counts is commonly secondary to medication or uremia. Primary platelet disorders are rare.

Platelet disorders caused by medications can cause bleeding whether affecting platelet function was the primary intent of the medication or a side effect. Some of the most common medications that can affect platelet function and cause a bleeding phenotype are clopidogrel, ticagrelor, and prasugrel, which inhibit P2Y12 (the ADP receptor) on platelets and impede platelet activation. Bleeding due to use of one of these agents may be detected on platelet aggregometry as a lack of aggregation in response to ADP. Aspirin and NSAIDs are cyclo-oxygenase 1 (COX1) and COX2 inhibitors, which in aggregometry will impair responses to stimulation by ADP, epinephrine, arachidonic acid, and low doses of collagen and thrombin, but not the major platelet agonists high-dose collagen and thrombin. Aspirin, as an irreversible inhibitor, will inhibit platelet function for 5 to 7 days, long after the unbound drug has been cleared. As such, bleeding exacerbated by aspirin use can be treated by transfusing platelets.

Several of the better characterized congenital platelet disorders are summarized in **Table 5**, although rare patients with abnormal aggregometry may have bleeding due to a platelet defect that is not yet known. In the past decade, genome-wide

Table 5
Genetic platelet disorders

Disorder	Gene/Protein Affected	Mechanism	Phenotype	Diagnosis
Glanzmann thrombasthenia	Glycoprotein IIb-IIIa (*GP2B, GP3A*)[24]	Impaired binding of platelets to fibrinogen	Mild to severe bleeding, petechiae, epistaxis	Aggregometry: impaired agglutination with all platelet agonists
Bernard Soulier	Glycoprotein 1b/IX (*GPIBA, GPIBB, GP9*)[25]	Impaired binding of platelets to von Willebrand factor	Mild to severe bleeding, may have thrombocytopenia	Aggregometry: impaired agglutination with ristocetin
Storage pool disorders	Hermansky-Pudlak (*HPS1*)[26] Chediack-Hidachi (*CHS1/LYST*)[27] Wiskott Aldrich (*WASp*)[28]	Impaired platelet activation due to dense platelet granule defects	Mucocutaneous bleeding, neutropenia, +/– albinism, pulmonary fibrosis	Often on the basis of other abnormalities, absence of dense granules on electron microscopy
Gray platelet syndrome	*NBEAL2,*[29] *GFI1B*[30]	Impaired platelet activation	Thrombocytopenia, large platelets, no alpha granules	Light and electron microscopy: absence of alpha granules
MYH9-related (eg, May-Hegglin anomaly)	*MYH9*[31]	Abnormal platelet cytoskeleton causing impaired clot retraction	Thrombocytopenia, large platelets, often moderate bleeding	Light microscopy: spindle-shaped inclusion bodies in neutrophils

Data from Refs.[24–31]

association studies found several additional variants, often in or near G protein coupled receptors, which may affect platelet function, leading to either gain or loss of function, although many of these variants have yet to be verified.[21–23] The congenital platelet disorders are often treated with transfusion of normal platelets, although patients lacking a complete complement of platelet antigens may mount an immune response to transfused platelets leading to platelet refractoriness.

SUMMARY

Accurate diagnosis of disorders of thrombosis and hemostasis require a thorough and directed history and physical examination, as well as specific testing, which can often be performed in a primary care setting. Although hemophilia was described in antiquity and has been a subject of research for over 200 years (Hay, NEJM 1813), in the past 50 years, with advances in laboratory testing, sequencing, and genome-wide association studies, there have been significant advances in our understanding of underlying mechanisms of disease, which has allowed development of specific clinical tests that both aid in characterization of the various disorders and provided a valuable tool in diagnosis.[32] Although a number of disease-causing and associated genes are known, a few of which have been discussed already, there are still many patients with a clinical bleeding phenotype for which we are unable to provide a specific diagnosis. With rapidly increasing availability of tools, such as next-generation sequencing and targeted arrays for discovering variants, we will surely be discovering more genes responsible for observed defects in hemostasis and with these discoveries will learn more about the mechanisms of disease and the diverse roles of our hemostatic machinery.[33]

REFERENCES

1. Chen VM, Hogg PJ. Encryption and decryption of tissue factor. J Thromb Haemost 2013;11(Suppl 1):277–84.
2. Furie B, Furie BC. Mechanisms of thrombus formation. N Engl J Med 2008;359(9): 938–49.
3. Rapaport SI, Rao LV. The tissue factor pathway: how it has become a "prima ballerina". Thromb Haemost 1995;74(1):7–17.
4. Morrissey JH, Choi SH, Smith SA. Polyphosphate: an ancient molecule that links platelets, coagulation, and inflammation. Blood 2012;119(25):5972–9.
5. Rodeghiero F, Castaman G, Tosetto A, et al. The discriminant power of bleeding history for the diagnosis of type 1 von Willebrand disease: an international, multicenter study. J Thromb Haemost 2005;3(12):2619–26.
6. Bowman M, Mundell G, Grabell J, et al. Generation and validation of the condensed MCMDM-1VWD bleeding questionnaire for von Willebrand disease. J Thromb Haemost 2008;6(12):2062–6.
7. Rodeghiero F, Tosetto A, Abshire T, et al. ISTH/SSC bleeding assessment tool: a standardized questionnaire and a proposal for a new bleeding score for inherited bleeding disorders. J Thromb Haemost 2010;8(9):2063–5.
8. Mauer AC, Khazanov NA, Levenkova N, et al. Impact of sex, age, race, ethnicity and aspirin use on bleeding symptoms in healthy adults. J Thromb Haemost 2011;9(1):100–8.
9. Nosek-Cenkowska B, Cheang MS, Pizzi NJ, et al. Bleeding/bruising symptomatology in children with and without bleeding disorders. Thromb Haemost 1991;65(3):237–41.

10. Onder O, Weinstein A, Hoyer LW. Pseudothrombocytopenia caused by platelet agglutinins that are reactive in blood anticoagulated with chelating agents. Blood 1980;56(2):177–82.
11. Ansell J, Hirsh J, Poller L, et al. The pharmacology and management of the vitamin K antagonists: the Seventh ACCP Conference on Antithrombotic and Thrombolytic Therapy. Chest 2004;126(3 Suppl):204S–33S.
12. Tripodi A, Mannucci PM. The coagulopathy of chronic liver disease. N Engl J Med 2011;365(2):147–56.
13. Mammen EF, Comp PC, Gosselin R, et al. PFA-100 system: a new method for assessment of platelet dysfunction. Semin Thromb Hemost 1998;24(2):195–202.
14. Cattaneo M, Cerletti C, Harrison P, et al. Recommendations for the standardization of light transmission aggregometry: a consensus of the working party from the Platelet Physiology Subcommittee of SSC/ISTH. J Thromb Haemost 2013; 11(6):1183–9.
15. Ruggeri ZM, Pareti FI, Mannucci PM, et al. Heightened interaction between platelets and factor VIII/von Willebrand factor in a new subtype of von Willebrand's disease. N Engl J Med 1980;302(19):1047–51.
16. Meyer AL, Malehsa D, Budde U, et al. Acquired von Willebrand syndrome in patients with a centrifugal or axial continuous flow left ventricular assist device. JACC Heart Fail 2014;2(2):141–5.
17. Tefferi A, Nichols WL. Acquired von Willebrand disease: concise review of occurrence, diagnosis, pathogenesis, and treatment. Am J Med 1997;103(6):536–40.
18. Franchini M, Gandini G, Di Paolantonio T, et al. Acquired hemophilia A: a concise review. Am J Hematol 2005;80(1):55–63.
19. Lusher JM, Arkin S, Abildgaard CF, et al. Recombinant factor VIII for the treatment of previously untreated patients with hemophilia A. Safety, efficacy, and development of inhibitors. Kogenate Previously Untreated Patient Study Group. N Engl J Med 1993;328(7):453–9.
20. Lazarin GA, Haque IS, Nazareth S, et al. An empirical estimate of carrier frequencies for 400+ causal Mendelian variants: results from an ethnically diverse clinical sample of 23,453 individuals. Genet Med 2013;15(3):178–86.
21. Johnson AD, Yanek LR, Chen MH, et al. Genome-wide meta-analyses identifies seven loci associated with platelet aggregation in response to agonists. Nat Genet 2010;42(7):608–13.
22. Qayyum R, Becker LC, Becker DM, et al. Genome-wide association study of platelet aggregation in African Americans. BMC Genet 2015;16:58.
23. Jones ML, Norman JE, Morgan NV, et al. Diversity and impact of rare variants in genes encoding the platelet G protein-coupled receptors. Thromb Haemost 2015;113(4):826–37.
24. Nurden AT, Fiore M, Nurden P, et al. Glanzmann thrombasthenia: a review of ITGA2B and ITGB3 defects with emphasis on variants, phenotypic variability, and mouse models. Blood 2011;118(23):5996–6005.
25. Savoia A, Pastore A, De Rocco D, et al. Clinical and genetic aspects of Bernard-Soulier syndrome: searching for genotype/phenotype correlations. Haematologica 2011;96(3):417–23.
26. Feng L, Novak EK, Hartnell LM, et al. The Hermansky-Pudlak syndrome 1 (HPS1) and HPS2 genes independently contribute to the production and function of platelet dense granules, melanosomes, and lysosomes. Blood 2002;99(5): 1651–8.
27. Kaplan J, De Domenico I, Ward DM. Chediak-Higashi syndrome. Curr Opin Hematol 2008;15(1):22–9.

28. Villa A, Notarangelo L, Macchi P, et al. X-linked thrombocytopenia and Wiskott-Aldrich syndrome are allelic diseases with mutations in the WASP gene. Nat Genet 1995;9(4):414–7.
29. Gunay-Aygun M, Falik-Zaccai TC, Vilboux T, et al. NBEAL2 is mutated in gray platelet syndrome and is required for biogenesis of platelet alpha-granules. Nat Genet 2011;43(8):732–4.
30. Monteferrario D, Bolar NA, Marneth AE, et al. A dominant-negative GFI1B mutation in the gray platelet syndrome. N Engl J Med 2014;370(3):245–53.
31. Althaus K, Greinacher A. MYH9-related platelet disorders. Semin Thromb Hemost 2009;35(2):189–203.
32. Lentaigne C, Freson K, Laffan MA, et al. Inherited platelet disorders: toward DNA-based diagnosis. Blood 2016;127(23):2814–23.
33. Simeoni I, Stephens JC, Hu F, et al. A high-throughput sequencing test for diagnosing inherited bleeding, thrombotic, and platelet disorders. Blood 2016;127(23):2791–803.

Transfusion Medicine

Nathan T. Connell, MD, MPH

KEYWORDS

- Transfusion medicine • Red cells • Platelets • FFP • Blood transfusion

KEY POINTS

- Transfusion of various blood components is indicated to correct abnormalities in oxygen carrying capacity or primary and secondary hemostasis.
- Various clinical tests can be used to ensure the compatibility between donor and recipient, although there are significant risks associated with transfusion.
- Risks of transfusion include transmission of infection, transfusion-related acute lung injury, transfusion-associated circulatory overload, and various hypersensitivity and hemolytic reactions.
- Adherence to the minimum number of units needed to reverse symptoms and avoidance of transfusion unless absolutely necessary will reduce the risks associated with transfusion.

INTRODUCTION

The practice of transfusion is to replace various components of the circulating blood system in order to alleviate symptoms or prevent complications due to the deficiency of a component, such as a coagulation factor or lack of platelets. With the exception of a few recombinant coagulation factors now available commercially, transfusion involves the practice of providing blood components obtained from human donors, as no viable synthetic transfusion product exists for most indications.

CLINICAL TESTS

Several tests are commonly used in the course of assessing the need for transfusion and the most appropriate donor unit to provide to the recipient. The decision to transfuse is often based on routine tests available in any laboratory, such as the complete blood count, indicating a low value of a particular cell line, such as red cells or platelets. Alternatively, specialized testing may show abnormalities in the coagulation or fibrinolytic system, which would require transfusion of fresh frozen plasma (FFP) or a derivative, such as cryoprecipitate.

Disclosure Statement: The author has nothing to disclose.
Division of Hematology, Brigham and Women's Hospital, Harvard Medical School, 75 Francis Street, Boston, MA 02115, USA
E-mail address: NTConnell@partners.org

One of the most commonly performed tests in the course of routine transfusion is the assessment of ABO type and screening for clinically significant alloantibodies. This test is commonly termed a *type and screen* and allows the transfusion service to start to narrow the choice of possible donor units. Although typing can be done to assess for a variety of red cell antigens, the most commonly performed is to look at ABO and Rhesus (or D antigen) compatibility. A sample is taken from the individual for whom the transfusion is intended and serum is separated from red cells. The serum is then mixed with red cells of known phenotype to assess for agglutination, which would suggest a significant antibody. Serum from patients with type A blood, for instance, will cause agglutination with red cells with B-antigen expression but not with A. Patients with type O blood will agglutinate with both A cells and B cells, as they have circulating antibodies to both of these antigens. Patients with type AB blood have tolerance to both antigens and, therefore, do not react to either A or B cells. Tests for blood type and antibody screening forms the basis for the concept of universal donors and universal recipients. Details of blood donor and recipient compatibility are outlined in **Table 1**.

In addition to determination of ABO type and Rhesus status, the serum is assessed for the presence of any clinically significant autoantibodies that may be present. These autoantibodies may form because of prior transfusion or pregnancy. The serum from the recipient is mixed with a panel of red cells of known phenotype. The pattern of agglutination across multiple panels allows the determination of whether a specific alloantibody exists in the intended recipient.

The direct antiglobulin test (DAT), commonly known as a direct Coombs test, is a more specific test and is not usually needed for routine transfusion practice. The test is designed to assess the presence of immunoglobulin G (IgG) or complement on the surface of patients' red cells (**Fig. 1**). A warm autoimmune hemolytic anemia will be DAT positive; the autoantibody may react with all potential donor cells, making crossmatch difficult.

INDIVIDUAL COMPONENT TRANSFUSION
Red Cells

Transfusion of red cell concentrate, sometimes referred to colloquially as packed red cells, is designed to increase the oxygen carrying capacity of the recipient due to the presence of anemia.

Table 1
Blood donor and recipient compatibility

ABO	Rh	RBC Transfusion		Plasma Transfusion	
		Donates to	Receives from	Donates to	Receives from
O	+	O+, A+, B+, AB+	O+, O−	O	O, A, B, AB
	−	O+, A+, B+, AB+, O−, A−, B−, AB−	O−		
A	+	A+, AB+	O+, A+, O−, A−	O, A	A, AB
	−	A+, AB+, A−, AB−	O−, A−		
B	+	B+, AB+	O+, B+, O−, B−	O, B	B, AB
	−	B+, AB+, B−, AB−	O−, B−		
AB	+	AB+	O+, A+, B+, AB+, O−, A−, B−, AB−	O, A, B, AB	AB
	−	AB+, AB−	O−, A−, B−, AB−		

Note: Rh matching is not necessary for plasma component transfusion.

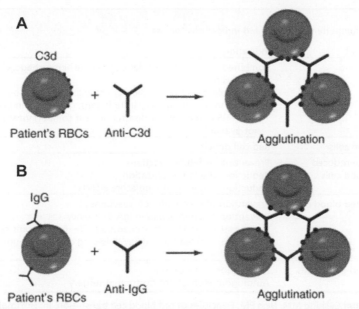

Fig. 1. DAT for detection of (*A*) erythrocyte-bound C3d or (*B*) IgG. Hemagglutination occurs when anti-C3d or anti-IgG can create a lattice structure by bridging sensitized red blood cells (RBCs). (*From* Ulrich J, Lechner K. Autoimmune hemolytic anemia. In: Hoffman RJ, Benz EJ, Silberstein LE, et al, editors. Hematology: basic principles and practice. 6th edition. Philadelphia: Elsevier; 2013. p. 617; with permission).

Various transfusion thresholds, across multiple types of clinical scenarios, have been studied; the current practice is to avoid the routine transfusion of red cells in asymptomatic unless patients have hemoglobin of less than 7 g/dL or equivalent hematocrit.[1] An acute drop in hemoglobin or onset of symptoms may warrant use of transfusion at higher thresholds. Some investigators have advocated for the use of a transfusion threshold of 10 g/dL in acute coronary syndromes, but further analysis of the data suggests this may be a practice with little evidence.[2,3] Patients undergoing chemotherapy often require periodic transfusions in order to maintain adequate red cell mass during decreased marrow production.[4] Patients with hemoglobinopathies may require ongoing transfusion depending on their underlying disorder and various other contributing factors. Those with beta-thalassemia major are typically transfusion dependent from childhood and require ongoing iron chelation in order to prevent complications, such as congestive heart failure and cirrhosis.[5] Those with sickle cell anemia may only require regular transfusions during the time of serious illness, such as the acute chest syndrome. Typically, mild cases can be treated with simple transfusion of 2 to 3 units of red cells, whereas moderate and severe cases may necessitate an exchange of patients' native red cells for donor red cells.[6] The use of simple transfusion in uncomplicated pain crisis is not routinely indicated.[7]

Various products are shown in **Table 2**. Donor red cells are separated from other blood components after collection and amount to approximately 300 mL of volume when added to their preservative solution. The presence of this solution allows longer storage times, up to 42 days by current standards.

Table 2	
Red cell component products and indications for use	
Component	Indications
Whole blood	Combined red cell/volume deficit (massive hemorrhage; exchange transfusion)
	Note: whole blood transfusion typically limited to resource-poor areas and certain military installations; guidelines in place for use in US civilian major disaster areas if component therapy is not available
Red blood cells	Red cell deficit
Leukocyte-reduced red blood cells	Prevention of febrile reactions
	Reduction of alloimmunization
	Reduction of immunomodulatory effects
Washed red blood cells	Prevention of severe allergic reactions
	Prevention of anaphylaxis in IgA deficiency
	Note: washed units = shortened shelf-life, labor intensive to produce, and lead to a delay in issuing compatible units for transfusion
Frozen red blood cells	Rare donor unit storage
	Autologous storage for postponed surgery

Adapted from Cushing MM, Ness PM. Principles of red blood cell transfusion. In: Hoffman RJ, Benz EJ, Silberstein LE, et al, editors. Hematology: basic principles and practice. 6th edition. Philadelphia: Elsevier; 2013. p. 1643; with permission.

Platelets

Platelets participate in primary hemostasis, and the bone marrow generally maintains a circulating platelet mass that is much higher than needed to provide adequate hemostasis. The typical platelet count runs between 150 and 400 $\times$ 10^9/L, but most individuals will tolerate much lower values. Current data suggest that the risk of bleeding does not increase in most situations until the platelet count is less than 50 $\times$ 10^9/L, under which trauma will lead to increased bleeding. Patients with a platelet count higher than this threshold can typically have general surgical procedures without any increased risk of bleeding as long as there are no other contributing factors such as drug-induced inhibition of platelets or deficiency of a coagulation factor.[8]

Platelets can be separated from donated whole units of blood or can be obtained from pheresis procedures to obtain them from a single donor. The platelets from a single unit of whole blood is not enough for a typical dose of transfused platelets and is usually combined with those of other donors and termed a pooled unit. Approximately 5 to 6 donors are pooled in order to achieve an adequate unit for transfusion. Usually, the number of platelets collected through apheresis techniques of a single donor is a sufficient quantity to transfuse and is termed a single-donor unit. The single-donor unit has the advantage of exposing recipients to a possible infection from only one donor but has the downside that if recipients have an antibody against the donor platelets, they may clear the entire transfused unit instead of just those platelets from one of the several donors in a pooled unit. Platelet units have a much shorter shelf-life of approximately 5 days. Additionally, the cooler temperatures used to store red cells causes platelet activation, so platelet units are stored at higher temperatures with periodic movement. Although these conditions extend the shelf-life of a unit of platelets, they also increase the risk of bacterial growth should the unit be contaminated.[9]

Platelet transfusion is indicated in several circumstances. For patients with severe thrombocytopenia and a platelet count less than 10×10^9/L, prophylactic transfusion is supported by evidence and guidelines from various professional societies, as this is the level at which the risk of spontaneous bleeding increases.[8,9] For platelet counts between 10 and 50×10^9/L, transfusion should usually only be considered if there is concomitant bleeding. Transfusion of platelets when the count is greater than 50×10^9/L is generally contraindicated, although certain situations may benefit. Patients with qualitative platelet defects, such as the congenital condition Glanzmann thrombasthenia, or acquired situations, such as aspirin inhibition, may benefit from transfusion of platelets regardless of the absolute platelet number should the clinical situation warrant.[10] Close discussion with a hematologist and transfusion medicine specialist is recommended.

Plasma

Transfusion of plasma is often indicated to address defects in the coagulation or fibrinolytic systems, and several products exist for clinical use.[11] The most commonly available product is FFP, which is separated from a whole unit of donated blood and usually frozen within 8 hours. The fact that the product is frozen means that it must be thawed before transfusion, which also means that the product is not as immediately available for transfusion as compared with red cells and platelets. Because almost the entire plasma volume of the donated unit is present, transfusion of FFP will provide all of the coagulation factors. The protein content is high, and rapid transfusion can lead to volume overload, so care must be taken when multiple units of FFP are given to patients in succession. In spite of this, FFP is not appropriate for volume expansion given the clinical efficacy of other available methods, such as normal saline infusion or red cell concentrate infusion in bleeding patients. When available and appropriate, use of prothrombin complex concentrates may allow the same correction in coagulopathy with significantly less volume.[12]

Transfusion of FFP is indicated in patients with abnormal coagulation profiles, such as prolongation of the prothrombin time (PT) with elevation of the international normalized ratio (INR) or prolongation of the partial thromboplastin time (PTT). The intrinsic INR of a unit of FFP ranges anywhere from 1.5 to 1.7, so transfusion of a unit of FFP is unlikely to bring patients' INR lower if they are already at this level.[13] Typically, transfusion should be limited to those patients whose INR is more than 2 before invasive procedures, although some proceduralists may advocate for a lower threshold in particularly high-risk procedures.[11] In patients with disseminated intravascular coagulation (DIC), FFP is often used to keep the PT and PTT less than 2 times the upper limit of the institution's normal limit for the respective laboratory's reference interval. Cryoprecipitate, also derived from plasma, is given in conjunction to address the coagulopathy that reduces from consumption of fibrinogen.[14,15]

Cryoprecipitate collected from the cooling of FFP in refrigerated conditions and has significant amounts of fibrinogen, coagulations factors VIII and XIII (FXIII), von Willebrand factor, and fibronectin. The indications for cryoprecipitate transfusion are typically replacement of these factors, such as in the need to increase fibrinogen in patients with a consumptive coagulopathy from DIC. Patients with FXIII deficiency often only need a single dose transfused given the long half-life of FXIII. Although cryoprecipitate has been used in patients with hemophilia A or von Willebrand disease, the availability of other specific plasma-derived and recombinant products has largely decreased the use of cryoprecipitate for these indications. Differences between the components in FFP and cryoprecipitate are outlined in **Table 3**.

Table 3
Volume and coagulation factors found in fresh frozen plasma and cryoprecipitate preparation

Product	Volume	Contains
FFP	200–250 mL	All coagulation factors present in the donor's blood
Cryoprecipitate	10–20 mL per unit and usually given as a pooled bag from multiple donors	Factor VIII, factor XIII, fibrinogen, fibronectin, von Willebrand factor

Plasma transfusion and therapeutic plasma exchange have a role in the treatment of certain disorders, such as thrombotic thrombocytopenic purpura (TTP). Although the absolute numbers of patients who undergo these treatments represent a small fraction of the total patients who receive plasma transfusion, the volume required by each patient with TTP represents a significant usage of the total plasma by many medical centers.[16] These procedures require the use of large-bore catheters in order to simultaneously remove native plasma and provide donor plasma.

Granulocytes

Granulocyte transfusion has had limited acceptance because of questions of efficacy and the complicated logistics in obtaining a sufficient number of granulocytes with rapid turnaround for infusion.[17] Unlike the minimal risk profile for donors of whole blood or apheresis platelet units, granulocyte donors must undergo growth factor stimulation in order to ensure enough cells can be obtained for infusion. These medications cause fatigue, bone pain, and fever. Additionally, there is a significant time burden on donors. The collected granulocytes require processing and only remain viable for a short period of time, typically less than 24 hours. Until future research shows clear efficacy, their use should be limited to a case-by-case basis for patients with refractory infections and profound neutropenia from either antineoplastic chemotherapy or hematopoietic stem cell transplant.

RISKS ASSOCIATED WITH TRANSFUSION

The transfusion of any blood product comes with risks of infection, hypersensitivity reactions, including anaphylaxis, and transfusion-related acute lung injury (TRALI). Additionally, there is a significant risk of volume overload, termed transfusion associated circulatory overload (TACO). TRALI and TACO can be very similar clinically, although other assessments of volume overload, such as jugular venous pressure and B-natriuretic peptide levels, can help distinguish the two.

Delayed hemolytic transfusion reactions may occur in patients who have a negative antibody screen on initial testing. These reactions are due to an amnestic response from the recipient's immune system due to a prior exposure. Antibodies to the Kidd antigen system are commonly implicated. The recipient's immune system recognizes the antigen on the donor red cells and rapidly begins to increase antibody production resulting in hemolysis of the donor red cells. This reaction typically occurs a few days after transfusion, although cases have been reported several weeks later. Repeat testing of the recipient will usually show a positive antibody screen. It is important to mark this finding in patients' transfusion history because the antibody may disappear again on repeat testing in the future, but they should not receive transfusion units from donors who have this antigen. Typically, supportive care is all that is needed, possibly with additional transfusion support depending on the speed of the hemolytic reaction.

Even without a delayed hemolytic reaction, patients may develop clinically significant alloantibodies to donor units, which restricts the number of future potential donors. The antibody screen should be repeated if even a few days have passed from the last transfusion to make sure that an alloantibody has not developed in the interim.

Some transfusion recipients are expected to require repeated transfusion in the future and are, therefore, more likely to develop alloantibodies if donor red cells are mismatched for minor RBC antigens. More extensive testing, such as an extended crossmatch, allows identification of the transfusion recipient's RBC phenotype to ensure that donor units are as closely matched as possible.

Predonation risk factor evaluation and rapid testing of units during postdonation processing have led to significant reductions in transfusion-associated infection. These methods, including nucleic acid testing, now mean the risk of a transfusion-associated viral infection, such as human immunodeficiency virus or hepatitis B/C, is approximately 1 in 1,000,000 or less.[18] Solvent/detergent processing of plasma products will inactivate many viruses. Bacterial infections are more common, particularly in platelet products, which cannot be stored at the colder temperatures used for red cell products.

The best treatment of any of the transfusion-associated risks is the initial prevention by restricting transfusion to those who have clear indications for such therapy, and only transfuse the minimum number of units necessary in those who are transfused. For those patients who start to experience a reaction while undergoing transfusion, the first and most important step is to stop the transfusion and assess the clinical scenario. Management is symptomatic. Patients may develop a rapidly progressive clinical deterioration that requires quick action, including administration of antihistamines, steroids, or diuretics to avoid acute respiratory failure. The blood bank should be immediately notified so various clerical checks are confirmed and testing started to evaluate the possibility of an error in crossmatching.

For patients suspected to have TRALI, supportive care should be initiated early. Oxygen supplementation needs to be administered to correct ongoing hypoxemia; mechanical ventilation through noninvasive or invasive methods may need to be used depending on the severity of patients' clinical situation. Institutional protocols for treatment of the acute respiratory distress syndrome should be followed along with hemodynamic support. The use of corticosteroids in TRALI is controversial and should be limited to patients in the first 14 days of their syndrome.

For those with suspected TACO, the treatment is similar to that of any cardiac overload syndrome. Supplemental oxygen should be administered to correct hypoxemia while diuretic therapy, such as furosemide, is initiated. A furosemide dose of 20 mg intravenously may be sufficient in diuretic-naïve patients, whereas higher doses may be necessary in those who are chronically receiving diuretic therapy for other indications. Frequent reevaluation with repeated doses of the diuretic may be necessary.

Fever can be due to hemolytic or nonhemolytic transfusions reactions. When a febrile hemolytic transfusion reaction occurs, it is most commonly due to transfusion of ABO incompatible blood. There is rapid hemolysis of the incompatible donor red cells with associated fever and dark urine. Patients may develop hypotension and require transient vasopressor support until the reaction finishes.

In contrast to the hemolytic transfusion reactions, a febrile nonhemolytic transfusion reaction is commonly due to the presence of transfused cytokines within the red cell unit. These cytokines come from donor leukocytes that break down during storage of the red cell unit. Many blood collection centers will use in-line filters to remove leukocytes during collection, as this is an effective way to reduce the risk of febrile nonhemolytic transfusion reactions. Alternatively, the unit may be leukoreduced during processing. Use of leukocyte filters at the time of transfusion is only marginally helpful in reducing the risk of febrile nonhemolytic transfusion reactions as the leukocytes have often disintegrated before transfusion but the inflammatory cytokines remain.

Questions often arise about how to prevent a transfusion reaction in someone who has previously reacted to a transfused unit. Most patients who react during a transfusion will not have similar reactions during subsequent transfusions as the reaction is related to the presence of a specific-donor antigen. By avoiding the transfusion of subsequent units from that donor, the risk of subsequent reactions is low. Patients with prior reactions should be closely watched during the subsequent transfusions in case of recurrence and prompt supportive measures initiated should another reaction occur.[19]

SUMMARY

The goal of transfusion is to alleviate symptoms or prevent complications due to deficiency of a blood component. Available transfusion units are obtained from volunteer donors who undergo an extensive screening process to manage the likelihood of an asymptomatic infection at the time of donation.

Transfusion should be limited to the minimum number of units necessary in order to limit the risks to the recipient. Routine red cell transfusion should be limited to those patients who have a hemoglobin less than 7 g/dL or those with symptoms from their anemia. Prophylactic platelet transfusion is indicated for those with a platelet count less than 10×10^9/L. Therapeutic platelet transfusion is considered for patients with active bleeding and a platelet count less than 50×10^9/L or patients with qualitative platelet defects and planned procedures. Plasma transfusion is indicated for correction of significant coagulopathies due to either congenital or acquired absence of one or more clotting factors. Each of the products has a role in the management of specific populations, and consultation with a hematologist or transfusion medicine specialist is recommended.

The best way to manage a transfusion reaction is to prevent it from happening in the first place. The first step in managing a suspected transfusion reaction is to stop the transfusion and initiate prompt supportive care while notifying the blood bank to initiate a transfusion reaction evaluation. Complications include infectious risks, transfusion-related acute lung injury, transfusion-associated circulatory overload, and both febrile and nonfebrile hemolytic transfusion reactions.

REFERENCES

1. Carson JL, Grossman BJ, Kleinman S, et al. Red blood cell transfusion: a clinical practice guideline from the AABB*. Ann Intern Med 2012;157(1):49–58.
2. Wu WC, Rathore SS, Wang Y, et al. Blood transfusion in elderly patients with acute myocardial infarction. N Engl J Med 2001;345(17):1230–6.
3. Shander A, Javidroozi M, Ozawa S, et al. What is really dangerous: anaemia or transfusion? Br J Anaesth 2011;107(Suppl 1):i41–59.
4. Schrijvers D. Management of anemia in cancer patients: transfusions. Oncologist 2011;16(Suppl 3):12–8.
5. Marsella M, Borgna-Pignatti C. Transfusional iron overload and iron chelation therapy in thalassemia major and sickle cell disease. Hematol Oncol Clin North Am 2014;28(4):703–27, vi.

6. Melton CW, Haynes J Jr. Sickle acute lung injury: role of prevention and early aggressive intervention strategies on outcome. Clin Chest Med 2006;27(3): 487–502, vii.
7. Hicks LK, Bering H, Carson KR, et al. Five hematologic tests and treatments to question. Blood 2014;124(24):3524–8.
8. Kaufman RM, Djulbegovic B, Gernsheimer T, et al. Platelet transfusion: a clinical practice guideline from the AABB. Ann Intern Med 2015;162(3):205–13.
9. Blumberg N, Heal JM, Phillips GL. Platelet transfusions: trigger, dose, benefits, and risks. F1000 Med Rep 2010;2:5.
10. Sarode R. How do I transfuse platelets (PLTs) to reverse anti-PLT drug effect? Transfusion 2012;52(4):695–701 [quiz: 694].
11. Roback JD, Caldwell S, Carson J, et al. Evidence-based practice guidelines for plasma transfusion. Transfusion 2010;50(6):1227–39.
12. Jones CA, Ducis K, Petrozzino J, et al. Prevention of treatment-related fluid overload reduces estimated effective cost of prothrombin complex concentrate in patients requiring rapid vitamin K antagonist reversal. Expert Rev Pharmacoecon Outcomes Res 2016;16(1):135–9.
13. Holland LL, Brooks JP. Toward rational fresh frozen plasma transfusion: the effect of plasma transfusion on coagulation test results. Am J Clin Pathol 2006;126(1): 133–9.
14. Levi M, Toh CH, Thachil J, et al. Guidelines for the diagnosis and management of disseminated intravascular coagulation. British Committee for Standards in Haematology. Br J Haematol 2009;145(1):24–33.
15. Thachil J, Falanga A, Levi M, et al. Management of cancer-associated disseminated intravascular coagulation: guidance from the SSC of the ISTH. J Thromb Haemost 2015;13(4):671–5.
16. Connell NT, Cheves T, Sweeney JD. Effect of ADAMTS13 activity turnaround time on plasma utilization for suspected thrombotic thrombocytopenic purpura. Transfusion 2016;56(2):354–9.
17. Vamvakas EC, Pineda AA. Meta-analysis of clinical studies of the efficacy of granulocyte transfusions in the treatment of bacterial sepsis. J Clin Apher 1996;11(1): 1–9.
18. Zou S, Stramer SL, Dodd RY. Donor testing and risk: current prevalence, incidence, and residual risk of transfusion-transmissible agents in US allogeneic donations. Transfus Med Rev 2012;26(2):119–28.
19. Tinegate H, Birchall J, Gray A, et al. Guideline on the investigation and management of acute transfusion reactions. Prepared by the BCSH Blood transfusion task force. Br J Haematol 2012;159(2):143–53.

Lymphoma

Emiliano N. Mugnaini, MD, PhD*, Nilanjan Ghosh, MD, PhD

KEYWORDS

- Lymphoma • Hodgkin • Non-Hodgkin • Diffuse large B cell • Follicular • Burkitt
- MALT • T cell

KEY POINTS

- Symptoms and signs suggestive of lymphoma include fevers, drenching night sweats, unintentional weight loss, lymphadenopathy, and splenomegaly.
- PET/computed tomography scans are the preferred modality for imaging in most lymphomas and can help with both staging and identifying biopsy site.
- Excisional lymph node biopsy is preferred over needle biopsy.
- Aggressive lymphomas need urgent evaluation and treatment. Burkitt lymphoma is an oncologic emergency and requires emergent hospitalization and initiation of treatment.
- Long-term complications of chemotherapy and radiotherapy should be recognized during follow-up.

The incidence of lymphoma in the United States from 2009 to 2013 was approximately 22 in 100,000 people, representing 5% of malignancies.[1] Median age at diagnosis is 63. Between the 1970s and1990s, incidence doubled, but it has been stable since. Overall survival (OS), fortunately, is improving, and is now estimated to be 72% at 5 years.[1] The understanding of lymphomas represents a challenge for many, owing to a large number of subtypes and complex terminology.

Lymphomas are divided into Hodgkin (HL), 10%, and non-Hodgkin (NHL), 90% (**Table 1**).[2] HL is further divided into classical and nonclassical types, and NHL into B-cell and T-cell and natural killer (NK) cell types. For clinical purposes, it is worthwhile to keep in mind whether a given lymphoma is aggressive (high grade) or indolent (low grade). Most indolent lymphomas are NHL (with the exception of nodular lymphocyte predominant HL). Traditionally, indolent lymphomas are less dangerous if left untreated, yet, at the same time they are more difficult to cure. Although this may seem paradoxic, it is because the lower proliferation rate of indolent tumors makes them less susceptible to chemotherapy. The aggressive or indolent nature of the

Disclosure Statement: The author has nothing to disclose (E.N. Mugnaini). Consultant for Celgene, Janssen, Abbvie (N. Ghosh).
Lymphoma Division, Department of Hematologic Oncology and Blood Disorders, Levine Cancer Center, Carolinas HealthCare System, 1021 Morehead Medical Drive, Charlotte, NC 28204, USA
* Corresponding author.
E-mail address: Emiliano.Mugnaini@carolinashealthcare.org

Table 1
Lymphoma subtypes with frequency

Lymphoma Subtype	Frequency (%)
Non-Hodgkin lymphoma	90
B-cell	
DLBCL	25–30
Follicular lymphoma	20
Extranodal marginal zone lymphoma of mucosa-associated lymphoid tissue	7
Chronic lymphocytic leukemia/small lymphocytic lymphoma	7
Mantle cell lymphoma	6
Burkitt lymphoma	1
Others	
Primary mediastinal large B-cell lymphoma	—
Primary effusion lymphoma	—
DLBCL associated with chronic inflammation	—
B-cell lymphoma, unclassifiable, with features intermediate between DLBCL and Burkitt lymphoma	—
B-cell lymphoma, unclassifiable, with features intermediate between DLBCL and classical HL	
ALK-positive large B-cell lymphoma	—
Intravascular large B-cell lymphoma	—
Primary cutaneous follicle center lymphoma	—
Lymphomatoid granulomatosis	—
Large B-cell lymphoma arising in HHV-8–associated multicentric Castleman disease	—
Plasmablastic lymphoma	—
Lymphoplasmacytic lymphoma	—
Splenic B-cell marginal zone lymphoma	—
Splenic B-cell lymphoma/leukemia, unclassifiable	—
Nodal marginal zone lymphoma	—
B-cell prolymphocytic leukemia	—
Hairy cell leukemia	—
T-cell/NK	9
Peripheral T-cell lymphoma, not otherwise specified	—
Angioimmunoblastic T-cell lymphoma	—
Extranodal NK/T-cell lymphoma, nasal type	—
Mycosis fungoides	—
Sézary syndrome	—
Anaplastic large-cell lymphoma, ALK positive	—
Anaplastic large-cell lymphoma, ALK negative	—
Enteropathy-type T-cell lymphoma	—
Hepatosplenic T-cell lymphoma	—
Subcutaneous panniculitis-like T-cell lymphoma	—
Primary cutaneous CD30+ T-cell lymphoproliferative disorders	—
Primary cutaneous peripheral T-cell lymphomas, rare subtypes	—

(continued on next page)

Table 1 (continued)	
Lymphoma Subtype	**Frequency (%)**
Epstein-Barr virus positive T-cell lymphoproliferative disease of childhood	—
T-cell prolymphocytic leukemia	—
Adult T-cell leukemia/lymphoma	—
T-cell large granular lymphocytic leukemia	—
Aggressive NK cell leukemia	—
Chronic lymphoproliferative disorders of NK cells	—
HL	10
Classical HL	10
Nonclassical HL	—

Abbreviations: DLBCL, diffuse large B-cell lymphoma; HL, Hodgkin lymphoma; HHV, human herpes virus; NK, natural killer.

Data from National Institute of Health, National Cancer Institute. Available at: www.seer.cancer. gov/statfacts/html. Accessed May 8, 2016; and Swerdlow SH, Campo E, Harris NL, et al. WHO classification of tumors of hematopoietic and lymphoid tissues. 4th edition. Lyon (France): IARC Press; 2008.

lymphoma, along with a given patient's performance status, will define whether treatment is curative, where survival is the goal, or palliative, where quality of life is determinate. With indolent lymphomas, where cure is not an option, the most important treatment may be to avoid overtreatment, *primum non nocere*, "above all else do no harm." Of note, nonaggressive, indolent lymphomas can transform over time into aggressive lymphomas. Such transformation, called Richter's transformation when from chronic lymphocytic lymphoma, may be diagnosed upon first presentation (already transformed) or later in previously diagnosed low-grade disease.

For any given case of lymphoma, usually no underlying etiology is identified. That being said, a number of environmental, infectious, and genetic factors predisposing to lymphoma have been identified. Occupational exposure risks include herbicides and pesticides (including, notably, Agent Orange). A number of infectious organisms are associated with specific lymphomas, including *Helicobacter pylori, Borrelia borgdorferi, Chlamydia psittaci,* and *Campylobacter jejuni.* Human T-cell lymphotropic virus can lead to development of adult T-cell leukemia/lymphoma. Hepatitis C has been associated with lymphoplasmacytic and marginal zone lymphomas, and human herpes virus-8 with primary effusion lymphoma and Castleman disease. Chronic stimulation itself may predispose to development of lymphoma. Enteropathy-associated lymphoma is defined by the presence of underlying inflammatory bowel disease. Chronic antigen exposure occurs with persistent infections such as Epstein-Barr virus (EBV) and cytomegalovirus. There is also an increased incidence of lymphomas in most immunodeficiency states, including infectious (human immunodeficiency virus), iatrogenic (transplant), or genetic (severe combined immunodeficiency). Extranodal NK/T-cell lymphoma, nasal type, is increased in Southern Asia and parts of Latin America. Certain drugs affecting the immune system, such as tumor necrosis factor-alpha inhibitors, have also been associated with an increased incidence of lymphoma, in particular T-cell lymphoma.

A diagnosis of lymphoma is obtained by tissue biopsy, most often this having been facilitated by the primary care physician. In order of increasing amount of material obtained, options for tissue biopsy include fine needle aspirate, core biopsy, incision/wedge biopsy, and excisional biopsy. Generally, the more tissue that can be obtained, the better. Indeed, the advantage of an excisional biopsy is that it allows for the assessment of whole lymph node architecture. When possible, it is best to obtain tissue where disease activity is greatest. PET/computed tomography (CT) scans, by measuring uptake of fluorodeoxyglucose, are an extremely useful indicator of the biologic activity of lymphoma.

The Ann Arbor Staging System (**Table 2**) was designed for HL, but is also used for NHL. The presence or absence of B symptoms, persistent fever, weight loss in excess of 10% of previous body weight over 6 months, or night sweats, are included in the staging for HL. Staging should be performed before the initiation of therapy. Basic blood work should include lactate dehydrogenase. Whole body PET/CT imaging is preferred over CT of the chest, abdomen, and pelvis for most lymphomas, with the exception of some low-grade lymphomas.[3] Bone marrow biopsy, with or without aspirate, is often performed for staging, but may be omitted for diffuse large B-cell lymphoma (DLBCL) and HL, because detection of stage IV over stage III disease with these lymphomas does not change treatment. In individual cases where a lymphoma is judged to be high risk, standard staging may be supplemented by cerebrospinal fluid testing.

The International Prognostic Index (IPI) was originally developed for diffuse DLBCL, but is used for most lymphomas.[4] Low IPI predicts a better outcome and high IPI a worse outcome (**Table 3**).[5] Further adaptation of the IPI may be found for specific lymphomas, for example, the FLIPI score for follicular lymphoma (FL) and the MIPI score for mantle cell lymphoma (MCL).

Antigen-specificity for B and T cells is defined by the cell-surface receptor, B-cell receptor or T-cell receptor, respectively. T cells are educated for antigen recognition in the thymus. B cells mature in the marrow and encounter foreign antigen for the first time within the lymph node germinal center (GC). As such, B cells may be divided into

Table 2 The Ann Arbor staging system	
Stage	**Definition**
I	Involvement of 1 lymph node region or lymphoid structure (eg, spleen, thymus, Waldeyer's ring)
II	Involvement of 2 or more lymph node regions/structures on the same side of the diaphragm
III	Involvement of 2 or more lymph node regions/structures on different sides of the diaphragm
IV	Involvement of extralymphatic sites beyond that designated as "E," including more than 1 extralymphatic involvement of any location or any involvement of bone marrow/liver
A	No B symptoms
B	Unexplained fever of greater than 38°C on 2 or more occasions within 1 mo, drenching night sweats within 1 mo, and/or unintentional weight loss 10% or more of body weight within 6 mo
E	Localized, solitary involvement of extralymphatic tissue (excluding bone marrow/liver)

From Lister TA, Crowther D, Sutcliffe SB, et al. Report of a committee convened to discuss the evaluation and staging of patients with Hodgkin's disease: Cotswolds meeting. J Clin Oncol 1989;7(11):1634–5.

Table 3 International prognostic index		
Risk Factors		
Age greater than 60 y		
Elevated lactate dehydrogenase		
Performance status 2 or higher (Eastern Cooperative Oncology Group) or 70 or greater (Karnofsky)		
Stage III or IV		
More than 1 extralymphatic site		
Risk Category	**No. of Risk Factors**	**4-y Overall Survival of Diffuse Large B-Cell Lymphoma (%)**
Low	0–1	91
Low-intermediate	2	81
High-intermediate	3	65
High	4–5	59

Adapted from Shipp MA, Harrington DP, Anderson JR, et al. A predictive model for aggressive non-Hodgkin's lymphoma. The International Non-Hodgkin's Lymphoma Prognostic Factors Project. N Engl J Med 1993;329:991; and Ziepert M, Hasenclever D, Kuhnt E, et al. Standard International Prognostic Index remains a valid predictor of outcome for patients with aggressive CD20+ B-cell lymphoma in the rituximab era. J Clin Oncol 2010;28:2377.

GC or post-GC. Post-GC, some B cells develop eventually into plasma cells, which secrete the soluble form of B-cell receptor, that is, immunoglobulin (Ig) or antibody. It is worthwhile to recall the physical structure of antibody, composed of 2 heavy and 2 light chains, each composed in turn of both variable and constant regions. It is the variable regions that determine antigen-specificity. For a given antibody, light chains may be of either kappa (κ) or lambda (λ) type. The most basic method for determining malignancy, or clonality, in B-cell lymphomas is by immunohistochemical (IHC) staining for light chains to demonstrate that a sample has lymphocytes expressing all kappa or all lambda light chains. This is referred to as light chain restriction and indicates the presence of a lymphocytic clone.

DIFFUSE LARGE B-CELL LYMPHOMA

DLBCL, an aggressive B-cell lymphoma, is the most common lymphoma, accounting for 25% to 30% of diagnoses (see **Table 1**). OS is about 60% at 5 years.[1] For most cases, no underlying etiology is identified. DLBCL arises most often within the lymph nodes, but presentation may also be outside of the lymphatic system, almost anywhere in the body. Indeed, DLBCL is the lymphoma most noted for extralymphatic presentation. The gastrointestinal tract is the most common site of extralymphatic presentation; testicular, ocular, and the central nervous system are other notable sites.

Histologic diagnosis includes the identification of areas of diffuse involvement by large lymphoid cells that stain positive for the B-cell marker CD20. Proliferation index, as determined by staining with the Ki-67 antibody, is expected to be moderate to high, albeit less than 100%.

Left untreated, survival in DLBCL is poor, but, fortunately, most DLBCL is chemosensitive. Treatment of DLBCL, therefore, is given with curative intent, performance status permitting. The gold standard for DLBCL treatment is R-CHOP (rituximab, cyclophosphamide, doxorubicin, vincristine, prednisone), with intravenous administration occurring over 1 day. It is given as an outpatient and repeated every 3 weeks.[6,7] In most cases, 6 cycles of systemic chemotherapy are given.[8] For very localized disease, combination chemoradiation therapy may be chosen, with just 3 cycles of systemic chemotherapy supplemented instead by local radiation with the purpose of limiting overall exposure to systemic chemotherapy (at the expense, of course, of radiation).[9] For patients with poor performance status, milder treatment options may include R-mini CHOP (with reduced doses of all drugs except rituximab), R-CHOP minus doxorubicin (R-CVP), or single-agent rituximab.

The primary side effects of R-CHOP include nausea, fatigue, malaise, hair loss, and cytopenias. These are generally well-managed and considered to be tolerable with appropriate supportive care, in particular antiemetic medications. In some patients, progressive peripheral neuropathy from vincristine may be limiting. Particular attention should be paid to cardiac comorbidities owing to the cardiac toxicity of doxorubicin, an anthracycline. A baseline echocardiography or multigated acquisition scan before initiation of chemotherapy is recommended. Granulocyte colony stimulating factor may be used to support the white blood cell count.

Reimaging by PET/CT is recommended to assess for treatment response at the conclusion of treatment. Reimaging is most often also performed during treatment, after 2 to 4 cycles of chemotherapy, with the purpose of identifying those cases not responding to initial chemotherapy. Patients who complete successful therapy should be followed at regular intervals for the possibility of disease recurrence. Follow-up consists of history, physical examination, and basic laboratory tests (cell counts, electrolytes, creatinine, liver function tests, lactate dehydrogenase). Repeat imaging is not needed routinely, in the absence of specific concerns. Most disease relapse occurs within 2 years, such that the follow-up interval is increased if the disease remains in remission beyond 5 years.

Clinical trials are currently underway assessing the efficacy and safety of adding immunomodulatory agents (lenalidomide)[10,11] or Bruton's tyrosine kinase inhibitors (ibrutinib)[12,13] to R-CHOP in previously untreated DLBCL.

For patients who do not respond or relapse after first-line chemotherapy, several salvage regimens are available. Common second-line regimens (eg, R-ICE, R-DHAP) are also generally well-tolerated, albeit somewhat more intense than R-CHOP, and will commonly require in-patient administration to administer the chemotherapeutic agents. Survival after successful salvage therapy for resistant/relapsed DLBCL is improved significantly if salvage therapy is followed by high-dose chemotherapy with autologous stem cell rescue (HD-SCT).[14] The advantage of HD-SCT lies in the high dose of the chemotherapy. A harvest of autologous peripheral blood stem cells before administration of high-dose chemotherapy allows for the use of doses so bone marrow toxic that they would otherwise kill the patient, were it not for rescue by stem cell reinfusion. In cases where second-line therapies fail, clinical trials or allogeneic stem cell transplantation may be indicated.

FOLLICULAR LYMPHOMA

FL, an indolent B-cell lymphoma, accounts for 20% of diagnoses, making it the second most common lymphoma (see **Table 1**). Median OS is 8 to 15 years, depending on extent of disease at diagnosis.[1] Presentation is most often with diffuse lymphadenopathy, but disease may also be localized or occasionally extralymphatic.

By definition, the cell of origin counterpart for FL is the follicular cell of the GC. In contrast with noncancerous follicular cells, in which the antiapoptotic protein Bcl-2 is downregulated (to allow for the cell turnover that occurs in the GC during an immune response), in FL cells, Bcl-2 is overexpressed. This overexpression is the result of translocation of the BCL-2 gene site (normally found on chromosome 18) to the B-cell receptor or Ig gene site (chromosome 14), namely t(14;18), found in almost all cases of FL. Like DLBCL therefore, FL is a GC-derived B-cell lymphoma. In some cases, FL may transform into DLBCL.

A histologic diagnosis of FL classically includes the identification within the lymph node of areas of considerable follicular proliferation and expansion. Within expanded follicules, in turn, small and large cells proliferate (just as in a reactive lymph node), but, rather than being a mix of B cells (CD20$^+$) and some T cells (CD3$^+$), in FL, the follicles are composed mostly of B cells positive for Bcl-2. There is, in FL, however, as in a reactive node, variation in actual size among follicle B cells, small cells called centrocytes and large cells centroblasts. The proportion of large cells, centroblasts, is reported as being either greater than, or less than, 15 cells per high-power field. The more large centroblasts, the higher the grade; in grades I and II there are 0 to 15 centroblasts per high-power field, whereas in grade III there are greater than 15 centroblasts per high-power field. The difference between FL grade IIIA and grade IIIB is the presence of a mixture of centrocytes and centroblasts in all follicles in grade IIIA versus the presence of follicles composed exclusively of centroblasts, immunoblasts (activated lymphocytes), or both, in grade IIIB. Of note, FL grade IIIB is managed as if it were DLBCL.

Prognosis in FL is predicted by the FLIPI score. As an indolent lymphoma, the clinical behavior of FL is variable. Some cases of FL remain asymptomatic, even untreated, or wax and wane on their own, whereas others progress and cause significant symptoms. Asymptomatic FL can be managed by watchful waiting, that is, monitoring for appearance of progression or significant symptoms before intervening. Median OS is measured in decades, such that often the diagnosis of FL does not impact life span. Treatment is generally not considered to be curative, so it must be chosen judiciously, weighing benefit against toxicities and keeping in mind that, after multiple therapies, toxicity will be cumulative. Some patients are uncomfortable with a watch and wait strategy because they feel that they are not receiving any treatment and will need counseling to understand that observation, in this case, is a form of treatment.

For localized FL confined to 1 lymph node area, radiotherapy may be chosen as the sole modality of therapy. More frequently, however, several areas within the body are involved in FL, and systemic therapy is needed. Often, a less aggressive approach, such as single-agent rituximab, may be chosen as first-line therapy, even for patients with good performance status, thus reserving the option of escalation in therapy for future need. For higher burden FL, it may be necessary to start with systemic cytotoxic chemotherapy. In FL, a number of different regimens have been used over the years. Since OS in FL is measured in decades, it has been difficult to demonstrate superiority of 1 regimen over another. Nevertheless, in recent years, rituximab-bendamustine (R-benda) has emerged as the most popular treatment, being superior to R-CHOP in terms of progression-free survival.[15] R-benda is usually given over 2 consecutive days as an outpatient, repeated every 4 weeks for 6 cycles. Side effects of this anthracycline-free drug are usually less than with R-CHOP, but leukopenia may be prolonged. Maintenance rituximab after completion of front-line systemic chemotherapy, usually once every 2 months for 2 years, has been shown to prolong progression-free survival but not OS.[16] As an incurable disease, relapse of FL is anticipated at some point, but can usually be treated with one of the other regimens available for frontline treatment. Upon recurrence of all indolent lymphomas, one should exclude the possibility of the transformation to aggressive lymphoma. In cases of early

FL relapse or other aggressive features, HD-SCT or allogeneic transplantation may be considered.

EXTRANODAL MARGINAL ZONE LYMPHOMA OF MUCOSA-ASSOCIATED LYMPHOID TISSUE

Normal mucosal tissue includes small lymphocytic aggregates dispersed in a noncontinuous fashion, known as mucosa-associated lymphoid tissue (MALT). These aggregates may proliferate during an immune response to form reactive follicles. Lymphoma that arises from the marginal zone of such aggregates is called MALT lymphoma, and accounts for about 7% of all lymphomas.[1] MALT lymphoma is an indolent B-cell lymphoma. OS survival is excellent, and there is less of a tendency to recur than with FL. Often disease is limited to local involvement, although multiple extranodal involvement and disseminated disease forms do exist. Repeated local antigen stimulation in the context of infections, autoimmune disease, or other inflammatory conditions may predispose to development of MALT. Well-documented associations include *H pylori* (gastric), *C psittaci* (ocular), *C jejuni* (small intestine), *B borgdorferi* (skin), as well as Hashimoto thyroiditis (thyroid) and Sjögren syndrome (salivary). Cell of origin is the marginal zone cell, a post-GC B-cell. Diagnosis is made by identifying aggregates of small lymphocytes with appropriate IHC staining profile (CD20$^+$ with a so-called null-phenotype, CD10$^-$ CD5$^-$).

In some cases, removal of the provocative agent may be sufficient treatment. In gastric MALT lymphoma, successful eradication of *H pylori* can often lead to full tumor regression, and this is therefore recommended as the first step in treatment (in cases of t(11;18) positive gastric MALT, *H pylori* eradication alone is insufficient).[17] An indolent disease, MALT lymphoma is treated with the same approach as discussed for FL, from watchful waiting to systemic cytotoxic chemotherapy, depending on the stage and clinical behavior.

MANTLE CELL LYMPHOMA

MCL, which comprises about 6% of lymphomas,[1] is often said to combine the worst characteristics of both the low- and high-grade lymphomas, namely, the incurability of low-grade lymphomas with the aggressive nature of high-grade lymphomas. Indeed, outcome for MCL is among the worst of all lymphoma subtypes; median OS is about 5 years.[1] That being said, MCL actually represents a wide spectrum of disease, with some patients, particularly elderly, who exhibit a very indolent course, allowing even just for observation without any treatment. The etiology is unknown, although there is a male predominance. MCL usually presents with widespread disease, most often with bone marrow involvement. Another common site of disease is the gastrointestinal tract. Multiple polyps, a condition known as lymphomatous polyposis, may cause gastrointestinal obstruction. Cell of origin, as the name suggests, is believed to be the mantle zone cell of the lymph node, that is, a post-GC B cell. The diagnosis is made by recognizing areas of small lymphoid cells, in some cases arising directly from an expanded mantle zone, with characteristic IHC staining and essentially always positive for cyclin D1, a protein involved in cell cycle regulation. The latter results from the translocation of the gene encoding for cyclin D1 on chromosome 11 and that encoding for Ig on chromosome 14, namely t(11;14). Prognosis in MCL is predicted by IPI score or, more selectively, by MIPI score.

Treatment for older patients with less aggressive disease may be with R-benda (or R-CHOP),[15] followed by maintenance rituximab.[18] Most patients, however, require more intensive regimens. One agent, cytarabine, is found in most regimens, because it has particular activity in MCL. Often, front-line chemotherapy is followed directly in first remission by consolidation with HDC-SCT. One such approach is the Nordic protocol (a maxi R-CHOP regimen alternating with rituximab-cytarabine).[19] Another regimen is alternating hyperCVAD (cyclophosphamide, vincristine, doxorubicin, dexamethasone) with methotrexate/cytarabine.[20] Lenalidomide and bortezomib have single-agent activity in relapsed MCL[21,22] and have recently been added to combination treatments for newly diagnosed MCL.[23,24] The Bruton's tyrosine kinase inhibitor, ibrutinib, has excellent activity in MCL and is approved by the US Food and Drug Administration for use in relapsed MCL.[25]

BURKITT LYMPHOMA

Burkitt lymphoma (BL) was first described by the Irish surgeon Denis Burkitt in 1958, and is a highly aggressive B-cell lymphoma. There are 3 forms of BL—endemic, spontaneous, and immunodeficiency associated. Endemic BL is the form recognized by Denis Burkitt while working as a missionary in Uganda and is a pediatric tumor typically presenting as a mandibular mass. It is the endemic form of BL that is most strongly associated with EBV infection; almost no cases occur in the absence of chronic infection. In North America, the most common form of BL is the spontaneous form. This form often presents as an abdominal mass. Immunodeficiency-associated BL is seen above all in human immunodeficiency virus infection; its presence, indeed, can be an AIDS-defining condition.

Molecularly, the pathogenesis of BL is driven by a translocation of the notorious cell proliferation protooncogene, C-MYC, to one of the sites encoding for Ig expression, either the heavy chain or one of the 2 light chains, κ or λ, respectively t(8;14), t(2;8), or t(8;22).

The diagnosis of BL is made by recognition of medium to large B cells with extremely high proliferation rate (Ki-67 essentially 100%), manifesting histologically as the classic starry sky appearance, a result of tingible-body macrophages with surrounding clearing.

BL should be approached as an oncologic emergency owing to a high proliferation rate of the tumor. This high proliferation rate necessitates immediate treatment with aggressive chemotherapy regimens in which the intensity of delivery is meant to outpace the capacity for cellular division to prevent development of tumor resistance. Failure to do so can result in rapid tumor proliferation, end-organ damage, and death. If treatment is initiated in a timely manner, however, results can be favorable. Treatment options for BL include R-hyperCVAD-methotrexate/cytarabine[26] and R-CODOX-M/IVAC (rituximab, cyclophosphamide, vincristine, doxorubicin, methotrexate/ifosfamide, etoposide, cytarabine).[27,28] Recently, DA-R-EPOCH, a regimen that is intense yet easier to tolerate than the others named, has shown promise.[29,30] With BL, obtaining a good response with the first attempt at treatment is considered to be of particular importance.

T-CELL LYMPHOMAS

T-cell and NK cell lymphomas include a diverse group of lymphomas that together account for only 10% of NHL, compared with the 90% that are B-cell lymphomas. It is only in recent years that T-cell lymphomas have been more reliably subtyped. The most frequently diagnosed T-cell lymphoma, however, remains the peripheral T-cell lymphoma not otherwise specified, a diagnosis of exclusion. Systemic chemotherapy used for T-cell lymphoma is in general similar to that used for aggressive B-cell NHL, save for the exception of rituximab (anti-CD20, a B-cell marker). Overall outcomes for

T-cell lymphomas are inferior to B-cell lymphomas. For CD30 positive T-cell lymphomas, an antibody–drug conjugate, brentuximab, has been effective.[31] Histone deacetylase inhibitors such as romidepsin and belinostat have modest activity in T-cell lymphoma.[32–34]

HODGKIN LYMPHOMA

HL accounts for 10% of lymphomas (see **Table 1**).[1] First identified by the British pathologist Thomas Hodgkin in 1832, HL is defined by the presence of pathologic Hodgkin Reed-Sternberg (HRS) cells, now known to be of B-cell origin. Similar to NHL, HL contains both aggressive and indolent forms, although classic HL, which is aggressive, accounts for 95% of cases. Morphologically, classical HL has been divided into 4 distinct variants, in decreasing order of frequency—nodular sclerosis, mixed cellularity, lymphocyte rich, and lymphocyte depleted. Today, however, all of the variants are managed similarly. Nonclassical HL, on the other hand, of which only 1 type exists—nodular lymphocyte predominant—is indolent and is managed differently, often with radiation only.

The incidence distribution of HL is bimodal. There is 1 age peak in the early 20s and a second in the mid 60s. For most cases, no underlying etiology is identified. In some subtypes of classical HL, a significant number of cases are positive for EBV, leading to speculation that EBV may play a causative role, but this remains to be proven. Some genetic predisposition to HL is suspected, because there is an increased relative risk among relatives of patients. Environmental factors are also suspected, with increased incidence among woodworkers, farmers, and meat processors. The incidence of HL is increased in patients with immunodeficiencies.

The primary care physician should be suspicious of young patients presenting with painless lymphadenopathy, with or without B symptoms. HL most often arises from within the lymph nodes, and frequently presents with B symptoms. The pattern of spread is often contiguous through successive lymph node stations. Some patients may complain of itching with no rash, and others of pain in involved lymph nodes after drinking alcohol. Histologically, the diagnosis of HL is made by identifying HRS cells, odd-looking large, bilobed cells often with 2 nuclei, appearing within a background of nonmalignant inflammatory cells. Determining B-cell lineage of the HRS cell was difficult, because IHC staining of several key markers in classical HL (CD20$^-$ CD30$^+$ CD15$^+$) is exactly opposite that expected for B cells. Left untreated, survival in classical HL is poor. Fortunately, however, most cases are highly chemosensitive and OS, at 86%, is very good.[1] Within the lymphoma field, HL is the showcase example of the effectiveness of modern chemotherapy.

Standard treatment in the United States and most other countries consists of ABVD (doxorubicin, bleomycin, vinblastine, and dacarbazine).[35,36] In Germany, the BEACOPP regimen (bleomycin, etoposide, doxorubicin, cyclophosphamide, vincristine, procarbazine, prednisone) has been popular.[37] Another regimen used is Stanford V (doxorubicin, vinblastine, mechlorethamine, vincristine, bleomycin, etoposide, prednisone).[38] Response rates to these regimens are similar, with BEACOPP giving slightly better cure rates than the other 2, but at the cost of a greater toxicity, including development of secondary acute myeloid leukemia/myelodysplastic syndrome, and, in particular, sterility, a side effect almost unseen with ABVD. In a relatively young population, sterility is naturally of major concern to patients.

ABVD requires intravenous administration over 1 day on alternate weeks, twice for each cycle. If disease is widespread (Ann Arbor stages III–IV), generally 6 cycles of ABVD are administered. For localized disease (Ann Arbor stages I–II), 2 to 4 cycles are usually preferred, depending on presence or absence of any unfavorable features: B symptoms, bulky mediastinal or greater than 10 cm disease, erythrocyte sedimentation rate of 50 or greater, or more than 3 sites of disease. Systemic chemotherapy may be supplemented by local radiation, either because of bulky disease or persistent PET/CT positivity after chemotherapy. Primary side effects of ABVD include a decrease in blood counts, nausea, malaise, fatigue, and hair loss, as well as peripheral neuropathy. These may be significant but can generally be managed acceptably. Baseline echocardiography or multigated acquisition are performed before initiation of treatment owing to the use of doxorubicin. Pulmonary toxicity of bleomycin is a concern, requiring baseline pulmonary function testing and monitoring for onset of any symptoms along the way.

Repeat imaging is recommended to assess for treatment response. HL is particularly PET/CT avid, so this modality is recommended. PET/CT results are judged by Deauville criteria, whereby signal less than (or equal to) the physiologic signal from the liver is negative (1–3) and signal greater than liver (4–5) is positive. Today, a strategy evolving in both the United States and Europe is to initiate treatment with ABVD, monitor response with repeat PET/CT after 2 cycles, and to escalate treatment to BEACOPP only for those patients with inadequate response.[39–44] Furthermore, recent indications are that if PET/CT response to ABVD is good, then bleomycin may be omitted from later cycles without compromising response, and sparing unnecessary pulmonary toxicity.[45]

Upon completion of therapy, patients require follow-up at regular intervals to exclude disease recurrence, again with only history and physical and basic laboratory tests, but without routine repeat imaging. Because many patients with HL are young and cured, they will live for a long time after treatment and must be monitored for late sequelae of treatment, in particular for the development of secondary cancers within previous radiation fields, such as lung, breast, or thyroid, as well as coronary artery disease.

For those patients with relapsed or resistant HL, several salvage regimens are available. Specifics are beyond the scope of this article, but 1 agent frequently preferred in this setting is brentuximab, a monoclonal antibody to CD30, one of the molecules for which HRS cells are distinctively positive, coupled to an antimitotic spindle apparatus agent, monomethyl auristatin. As of today, brentuximab is approved by the US Food and Drug Administration for HL as a second-line agent only,[46] but trials are underway using brentuximab upfront in ABVD, in place of bleomycin.[47] Salvage therapy in HL, if successful, may be followed by consolidation with HD-SCT. Where disease is fully resistant or relapses again after HD-SCT, experimental agents within the context of a clinical trial are indicated, or, in selected cases, allogeneic stem cell transplantation. Nivolumab and pembrolizumab, programmed death-1 inhibitors, have shown remarkable overall response rates (up to 87%) in refractory HL in phase I trials.[48–50]

SUMMARY

It is important for the primary care clinician to recognize the symptoms and signs that are suggestive of lymphoma: fevers, drenching night sweats, unintentional weight loss, lymphadenopathy, and splenomegaly. Diagnosis of lymphoma is made on biopsy. Excisional biopsy is preferred because it allows for examination of whole lymph node architecture. Lymphomas may be grouped into NHL and HL. Treatment options of chemotherapy and radiotherapy vary by histologic subtype. Clinically, the most important distinction is to recognize whether a given lymphoma is of an indolent or aggressive nature. Aggressive lymphomas are more dangerous if left untreated, yet, a higher cell proliferation rate renders them more chemosensitive. As such, aggressive lymphomas are managed with curative intent, and need urgent evaluation and treatment. Indolent lymphomas, in contrast, are in general incurable, so quality of life must be balanced against toxicity of treatment when determining if and how to treat them.

ACKNOWLEDGMENTS

The authors thank Jared Block, MD, Department of Pathology and Laboratory Medicine, for a careful and insightful review of the article.

REFERENCES

1. National Institute of Health, National Cancer Institute. Cancer stat fact sheets. Available at: www.seer.cancer.gov/statfacts/html. Accessed May 8, 2016.
2. Swerdlow SH, Campo E, Harris NL, et al. WHO classification of tumors of hematopoietic and lymphoid tissues. 4th edition. Lyon (France): IARC Press; 2008.
3. Elstrom R, Guan L, Baker G, et al. Utility of FDG-PET scanning in lymphoma by WHO classification. Blood 2003;101(10):3875–6.
4. Shipp MA, Harrington DP, Anderson JR, et al. A predictive model for aggressive non-Hodgkin's lymphoma. The International Non-Hodgkin's lymphoma prognostic factors project. N Engl J Med 1993;329:987–94.
5. Ziepert M, Hasenclever D, Kuhnt E, et al. Standard International Prognostic Index remains a valid predictor of outcome for patients with aggressive CD20+ B-cell lymphoma in the rituximab era. J Clin Oncol 2010;28:2373–80.
6. Coiffier B, Lepage E, Briere J, et al. CHOP chemotherapy plus rituximab compared with CHOP alone in elderly patients with diffuse large-B-cell lymphoma. N Engl J Med 2002;346(4):235–42.
7. Coiffier B, Thieblemont C, Van Den Neste E, et al. Long-term outcome of patients in the LNH-98.5 trial, the first randomized study comparing rituximab-CHOP to standard CHOP chemotherapy in DLBCL patients: a study by the Groupe d'Etudes des Lymphomes de l'Adulte. Blood 2010;116(12):2040–5.
8. Pfreundschuh M, Schubert J, Ziepert M, et al. Six versus eight cycles of bi-weekly CHOP-14 with or without rituximab in elderly patients with aggressive CD20+ B-cell lymphomas: a randomised controlled trial (RICOVER-60). Lancet Oncol 2008;9:105–16.
9. Persky DO, Unger JM, Spier CM, et al. Phase II study of rituximab plus three cycles of CHOP and involved-field radiotherapy for patients with limited-stage aggressive B-cell lymphoma: Southwest Oncology Group study 0014. J Clin Oncol 2008;26(14):2258–63.
10. Nowakowski GS, LaPlant B, Macon WR, et al. Lenalidomide combined with R-CHOP overcomes negative prognostic impact of non-germinal center B-cell phenotype in newly diagnosed diffuse large B-Cell lymphoma: a phase II study. J Clin Oncol 2015;33(3):251–7.
11. Grzegorz S, Nowakowski GS, Chiappella A, et al. Randomized, phase III trial of the efficacy and safety of lenalidomide plus R-CHOP vs R-CHOP in patients with untreated ABC-type diffuse large B-cell lymphoma (DLC002; NCT02285062). American Society of Clinical Oncology Annual Meeting. Chicago, May 29 – June 2, 2015, [abstract: TPS8600].
12. Younes A, Thieblemont C, Morschhauser F, et al. Combination of ibrutinib with rituximab, cyclophosphamide, doxorubicin, vincristine, and prednisone (R-CHOP)

for treatment-naive patients with CD20-positive B-cell non-Hodgkin lymphoma: a non-randomised, phase 1b study. Lancet Oncol 2014;15(9):1019–26.

13. Wilson WH, Young RM, Schmitz R, et al. Targeting B cell receptor signaling with ibrutinib in diffuse large B cell lymphoma. Nat Med 2015;21(8):922–6.

14. Philip T, Guglielmi C, Hagenbeek A, et al. Autologous bone marrow transplantation as compared with salvage chemotherapy in relapses of chemotherapy-sensitive non-Hodgkin's lymphoma. N Engl J Med 1995;333(23):1540–5.

15. Rummel MJ, Niederle N, Maschmeyer G, et al. Bendamustine plus rituximab versus CHOP plus rituximab as first-line treatment for patients with indolent and mantle-cell lymphomas: an open-label, multicentre, randomised, phase 3 non-inferiority trial. Lancet 2013;381(9873):1203–10.

16. Salles G, Seymour JF, Offner F, et al. Rituximab maintenance for 2 years in patients with high tumour burden follicular lymphoma responding to rituximab plus chemotherapy (PRIMA): a phase 3, randomized controlled trial. Lancet 2010;377:42–51.

17. Nakamura S, Sugiyama T, Matsumoto T, et al. Long-term clinical outcome of gastric MALT lymphoma after eradication of Helicobacter pylori: a multicentre cohort follow-up study of 420 patients in Japan. Gut 2012;61(4):507–13.

18. Kluin-Nelemans HC, Hoster E, Hermine O, et al. Treatment of older patients with mantle-cell lymphoma. N Engl J Med 2012;367(6):520–31.

19. Geisler CH, Kolstad A, Laurell A, et al. Long-term progression-free survival of mantle cell lymphoma after intensive front-line immunochemotherapy with in vivo-purged stem cell rescue: a nonrandomized phase 2 multicenter study by the Nordic Lymphoma Group. Blood 2008;112(7):2687–93.

20. Romaguera JE, Fayad L, Rodriguez MA, et al. High rate of durable remissions after treatment of newly diagnosed aggressive mantle-cell lymphoma with rituximab plus hyper-CVAD alternating with rituximab plus high-dose methotrexate and cytarabine. J Clin Oncol 2005;23(28):7013–23.

21. Goy A, Sinha R, Williams ME, et al. Single-agent lenalidomide in patients with mantle-cell lymphoma who relapsed or progressed after or were refractory to bortezomib: phase II MCL-001 (EMERGE) study. J Clin Oncol 2013;31(29):3688–95.

22. Fisher RI, Bernstein SH, Kahl BS, et al. Multicenter phase II study of bortezomib in patients with relapsed or refractory mantle cell lymphoma. J Clin Oncol 2006; 24(30):4867–74.

23. Ruan J, Martin P, Shah B, et al. Lenalidomide plus Rituximab as Initial Treatment for Mantle-Cell Lymphoma. N Engl J Med 2015;373(19):1835–44.

24. Robak T, Huang H, Jin J, et al. Bortezomib-based therapy for newly diagnosed mantle-cell lymphoma. N Engl J Med 2015;372(10):944–53.

25. Wang ML, Rule S, Martin P, et al. Targeting BTK with ibrutinib in relapsed or refractory mantle-cell lymphoma. N Engl J Med 2013;369(6):507–16.

26. Thomas DA, Faderl S, O'Brien S, et al. Chemoimmunotherapy with hyper-CVAD plus rituximab for the treatment of adult Burkitt and Burkitt-type lymphoma or acute lymphoblastic leukemia. Cancer 2006;106(7):1569–80.

27. Magrath I, Adde M, Shad A, et al. Adults and children with small noncleaved-cell lymphoma have a similar excellent outcome when treated with the same chemotherapy regimen. J Clin Oncol 1996;14:925–34.

28. Barnes JA, Lacasce AS, Feng Y, et al. Evaluation of the addition of rituximab to CODOX-M/IVAC for Burkitt's lymphoma: a retrospective analysis. Ann Oncol 2011;22:1859–64.

29. Dunleavy K, Pittaluga S, Shovlin M, et al. Low-intensity therapy in adults with Burkitt's lymphoma. N Engl J Med 2013;369(20):1915–25.

30. Dunleavy K, Noy A, Abramson JS, et al. Risk-adapted therapy in adults with Burkitt lymphoma: preliminary report of a multicenter prospective phase II study of DA-EPOCH-R. American Society of Hematology Annual Meeting. Orlando, December 5–8, 2015, [abstract: 342].

31. Pro B, Advani R, Brice P, et al. Brentuximab vedotin (SGN-35) in patients with relapsed or refractory systemic anaplastic large-cell lymphoma: results of a phase II study. J Clin Oncol 2012 Jun 20;30(18):2190–6.

32. Piekarz RL, Frye R, Prince HM, et al. Phase 2 trial of romidepsin in patients with peripheral T-cell lymphoma. Blood 2011;117(22):5827–34.

33. Coiffier B, Pro B, Prince HM, et al. Results from a pivotal, open-label, phase II study of romidepsin in relapsed or refractory peripheral T-cell lymphoma after prior systemic therapy. J Clin Oncol 2012;30(6):631–6.

34. O'Connor OA, Horwitz S, Masszi T, et al. Belinostat in patients with relapsed or refractory peripheral T-Cell Lymphoma: results of the pivotal phase II BELIEF (CLN-19) study. J Clin Oncol 2015;33(23):2492–9.

35. Bonadonna G, Zucali R, Monfardini S, et al. Combination chemotherapy of Hodgkin's disease with adriamycin, bleomycin, vinblastine, and imidazole carboxamide versus MOPP. Cancer 1975;36(1):252–9.

36. Bonadonna G, Valagussa P, Santoro A. Alternating non-cross-resistant combination chemotherapy or MOPP in stage IV Hodgkin's disease. a report of 8-year results. Ann Intern Med 1986;104(6):739–46.

37. Diehl V, Franklin J, Pfreundschuh M, et al. Standard and increased-dose BEACOPP chemotherapy compared with COPP-ABVD for advanced Hodgkin's disease. N Engl J Med 2003;348(24):2386–95.

38. Horning SJ, Hoppe RT, Breslin S, et al. Stanford V and radiotherapy for locally extensive and advanced Hodgkin's disease: mature results of a prospective clinical trial. J Clin Oncol 2002;20(3):630–7.

39. Press OW, Li H, Schöder H, et al. US Intergroup trial of response-adapted therapy for stage III to IV Hodgkin lymphoma using early interim fluorodeoxyglucose-positron emission tomography imaging: Southwest Oncology Group S0816. J Clin Oncol 2016;34(17):2020–7.

40. Radford J, Illidge T, Counsell N, et al. Results of a trial of PET-directed therapy for early-stage Hodgkin's lymphoma. N Engl J Med 2015;372(17):1598–607.

41. Straus DJ, Pitcher B, Kostakoglu L, et al. Initial results of US intergroup trial of response-adapted chemotherapy or chemotherapy/radiation therapy based on PET for non-bulky stage I and II Hodgkin lymphoma (CALGB/Alliance 50604). American Society of Hematology Annual Meeting. Orlando, December 5–8, 2015, [abstract: 578].

42. Raemaekers J. Early FDG-PET adapted treatment improves the outcome of early FDG-PET-positive patients with stages I/II Hodgkin lymphoma (HL): final results of the randomized intergroup EORTC/LYSA/FIL H10 trial. 13th International Conference on Malignant Lymphoma, Lugano (Switzerland), June 17–20, 2015, Late-Breaking Abstract.

43. Gallamini A, Rossi A, Patti C, et al. Interim PET-adapted chemotherapy in advanced Hodgkin lymphoma. Results of the second interim analysis of the Italian GITIL/FIL DH0607 trial. 13th International Conference on Malignant Lymphoma, Lugano (Switzerland), June 17–20, 2015, [abstract: 118].

44. Barrington SF, Kirkwood AA, Franceschetto A, et al. PET-CT for staging and early response: results from the Response-Adapted Therapy in Advanced Hodgkin Lymphoma study. Blood 2016;127(12):1531–8.

45. Johnson PW, Federico M, Fosså A, et al. Response-adapted therapy based on interim FDG-PET scans in advanced Hodgkin lymphoma: first analysis of the safety of de-escalation and efficacy of escalation in the international RATHL Study (CRUK/07/033). 13th International Conference on Malignant Lymphoma, Lugano (Switzerland), June 17–20, 2015, [abstract: 008].
46. Younes A, Gopal AK, Smith SE, et al. Results of a pivotal phase II study of brentuximab vedotin for patients with relapsed or refractory Hodgkin's lymphoma. J Clin Oncol 2012;30(18):2183–9.
47. Younes A, Connors JM, Park SI, et al. Brentuximab vedotin combined with ABVD or AVD for patients with newly diagnosed Hodgkin's lymphoma: a phase 1, open-label, dose-escalation study. Lancet Oncol 2013;14(13):1348–56.
48. Ansell SM, Lesokhin AM, Borrello I, et al. PD-1 blockade with nivolumab in relapsed or refractory Hodgkin's lymphoma. N Engl J Med 2015;372(4):311–9.
49. Ansell S, Armand P, Timmerman JM, et al. Nivolumab in patients with relapsed or refractory classical Hodgkin lymphoma: clinical outcomes from extended follow-up of a Phase 1 study (CA209–039). American Society of Hematology Annual Meeting. Orlando, December 5–8, 2015, [abstract: 583].
50. Armand P, Shipp MA, Ribrag V, et al. PD-1 blockade with pembrolizumab in patients with classical Hodgkin lymphoma after brentuximab vedotin failure: safety, efficacy, and biomarker assessment. American Society of Hematology Annual Meeting. Orlando, December 5–8, 2015, [abstract: 584].

Plasma Cell Disorders

Jorge J. Castillo, MD

KEYWORDS

- MGUS • Multiple myeloma • Waldenström macroglobulinemia • Amyloidosis
- POEMS

KEY POINTS

- Monoclonal gammopathy of undetermined significance is a premalignant condition with an incidence of 3% in the general population and a rate of progression to myeloma of 1% per year.
- Myeloma patients can present with anemia, bone lesions, renal dysfunction, and/or hypercalcemia. There are now multiple treatment options for myeloma, which have improved survival.
- Waldenström macroglobulinemia can present with anemia, hyperviscosity, and/or neuropathy. The US Food and Drug Administration has approved ibrutinib to treat Waldenström macroglobulinemia.
- Polyneuropathy, organomegaly, endocrinopathy, monoclonal protein, and skin changes syndrome is a rare disease with a prolonged survival but high rates of disability due to progressive neuropathy.

INTRODUCTION

Plasma cell disorders are a heterogeneous group of blood disorders characterized by the detection of a monoclonal paraprotein in the serum or urine and/or the presence of monoclonal plasma cells in the bone marrow space or, rarely, in other tissues. Plasma cell diseases include monoclonal gammopathy of undetermined significance (MGUS), multiple myeloma (MM), lymphoplasmacytic lymphoma/Waldenström macroglobulinemia (LPL/WM), amyloidosis, and POEMS syndrome (Polyneuropathy, Organomegaly, Endocrinopathy, Monoclonal protein, and Skin changes).

MONOCLONAL GAMMOPATHY OF UNDETERMINED SIGNIFICANCE

MGUS is a clinically asymptomatic premalignant clonal plasma cell, and in some cases, lymphoplasmacytic disorder that is typically identified incidentally while patients are being worked up for other reasons, such as anemia, neuropathy, or hypercalcemia, among others.

Disclosure Statement: Advisory Board: Pharmacyclics, Alexion. Consultancy: Biogen Idec, Otsuka. Honoraria: Celgene, Janssen. Research Funding: Abbvie, Gilead, Millennium, Pharmacyclics.
Division of Hematological Malignancies, Dana-Farber Cancer Institute, Harvard Medical School, 450 Brookline Avenue, Mayer 221, Boston, MA 02215, USA
E-mail address: Jorgej_castillo@dfci.harvard.edu

MGUS has been identified in 1% to 2% of individuals in studies from the United States and Europe.[1–3] The incidence and prevalence of MGUS increase with age, are higher in men than women, and are higher in individuals of African descent.[4,5] Limited data suggest the incidence of MGUS in Asians and Hispanics is lower than in Caucasians.[6,7] First-degree relatives of patients with MGUS have a higher risk of developing other plasma cell disorders.[8,9]

Current population-based data support that about half of individuals diagnosed with MGUS at age 70 had had a monoclonal paraprotein for 10 years.[10] Patients are typically diagnosed due to the presence of a monoclonal paraprotein in serum or urine protein electrophoresis (SPEP and UPEP, respectively). Immunoglobulin G (IgG) MGUS is the most common type (70% of the cases), followed by IgM (15%) and IgA (12%).[11] IgD, IgE, and light chain–only MGUS have been reported.

The diagnosis of MGUS is made when a monoclonal paraprotein less than 3 g/dL is found in an asymptomatic patient. The minimum initial evaluation for patients with MGUS should include the following:

- Complete blood count (CBC)
- Serum calcium and creatinine levels
- SPEP/UPEP with immunofixation
- Serum free light chain (FLC) levels and ratio
- Quantitation of immunoglobulins
- Skeletal survey (radiographs)

A bone marrow biopsy is indicated in patients with an IgG monoclonal paraprotein greater than or equal to 1.5 g/dL, patients with non-IgG (IgM, IgA, IgD, light chain–only) monoclonal paraprotein of any size, patients with an abnormal FLC ratio, and in patients with abnormalities of the CBC, creatinine, calcium, or radiographs. Therefore, a bone marrow biopsy can be deferred in patients with IgG MGUS with monoclonal protein less than 1.5 g/dL, normal FLC ratio, and with no clinical concerns for myeloma. In patients with IgM MGUS, computed tomography (CT) scans should be considered to evaluate for the presence of lymphadenopathy and/or hepatosplenomegaly.

The diagnostic criteria for MGUS are as follows[12]:

Diagnostic criteria for non-IgM MGUS
- Presence of a serum monoclonal protein (IgG, IgA, or IgD) less than 3 g/dL
- Fewer than 10% clonal plasma cells in the bone marrow
- Absence of lytic bone lesions, anemia, hypercalcemia, and renal insufficiency related to the plasma cell disorder.

Diagnostic criteria for IgM MGUS
- Presence of a serum IgM monoclonal protein less than 3 g/dL.
- Fewer than 10% clonal plasma cells in the bone marrow
- Absence of anemia, constitutional symptoms, hyperviscosity, lymphadenopathy, hepatomegaly, or splenomegaly related to the plasma cell disorder

Diagnostic criteria for light chain MGUS
- Abnormal FLC ratio (ie, kappa to lambda ratio <0.26 or >1.65)
- Increased level of the appropriate involved light chain
- No monoclonal immunoglobulin heavy chain (IgG, IgA, IgD, or IgM)
- Fewer than 10% clonal plasma cells in the bone marrow
- Absence of lytic bone lesions, anemia, hypercalcemia, and renal insufficiency related to the plasma cell disorder

Each of the clinical types of MGUS carries a risk of progressing to a malignant plasma cell or lymphoplasmacytic disorder of about 1% per year. It is impossible, however, to know with certainty which patient will have a benign course and which patient will eventually progress. Therefore, patients with MGUS should be monitored for progression and potential complications.

Patients with non-IgM MGUS might progress into MM, and in smaller proportion into AL amyloidosis, light chain deposition disease, and other lymphoproliferative disorders.[11] Patients with IgM MGUS can progress into WM, and rarely, into AL amyloidosis or IgM MM.[13] Light chain MGUS can progress into light chain MM, AL amyloidosis, or light chain deposition disease.[14]

Three risk factors are currently used for evaluating the risk of progression from MGUS to symptomatic plasma cell or lymphoplasmacytic disorder[15,16]:

- Serum monoclonal paraprotein level greater than or equal to 1.5 g/dL
- Non-IgG MGUS
- Abnormal serum FLC ratio

The 20-year risk of progression is as follows[17]:

- 3 risk factors (high risk): 58%
- 2 risk factors (high-intermediate risk): 37%
- 1 risk factor (low-intermediate risk): 21%
- 0 risk factors (low risk): 5%

Patients with low-risk MGUS can be followed with history and physical and routine laboratory studies on a yearly basis. All other patients should be followed with at least an annual examination, CBC, calcium and creatinine levels, SPEP/UPEP, and serum FLC ratio. Additional investigation should be undertaken if any of the following develop:

- Bone pain
- Fatigue or generalized weakness
- Constitutional symptoms (unintentional weight loss, fever, night sweats)
- Neurologic symptoms (neuropathy, headache, dizziness)
- Bleeding
- Symptoms suggestive of amyloidosis (macroglossia, nephrotic syndrome, restrictive cardiomyopathy)
- Lymphadenopathy, hepatomegaly, or splenomegaly
- Abnormal laboratory findings (anemia, elevated creatinine, hypercalcemia)

The survival of patients with MGUS approximates the survival of the general population.[18] Patients with MGUS, however, have a higher risk of fractures, thromboembolic episodes, and secondary myeloid malignancies.[19-24] Patients with MGUS should undergo bone densitometry studies and receive bisphosphonates if there is evidence of osteopenia or osteoporosis.

MULTIPLE MYELOMA

MM is a plasma cell neoplasm characterized by the accumulation of malignant plasma cells in the bone marrow producing a monoclonal paraprotein. A diagnosis of MM should be suspected in these following scenarios:

- Unexplained anemia
- Hypercalcemia
- Acute renal failure or nephrotic syndrome

- Bone fractures or presence of bone lytic lesions on imaging studies
- Increased serum protein or presence of monoclonal paraprotein in serum or urine

MM accounts for 10% of all hematologic malignancies with an incidence that has remained stable for the last 5 decades.[25,26] The median age at diagnosis is 66 years with 10% of patients being younger than 50 years, and a slight male predominance.[27] The risk of MM is higher in blacks than in whites, and lower in Asians and Mexicans.[28,29] Individuals with a first-degree family member with MM have a 4-fold increased risk of developing MM.[30]

The most common presenting signs and symptoms of MM include the following:

- Anemia (75%), typically normochromic and normocytic
- Bone pain (60%), particularly back and chest
- Elevated creatinine (50%), typically associated with light chain cast nephropathy (myeloma kidney), amyloid kidney, or light chain deposition disease
- Hypercalcemia (30%), which should be treated emergently if calcium greater than or equal to 11 mg/dL
- Fatigue (30%)
- Weight loss (25%)

Less common signs or symptoms of MM include neuropathy (5%), hepatosplenomegaly (5%), lymphadenopathy (1%), and fever (1%).

Cord compression due to plasmacytoma or vertebral fracture may be seen in 5% of patients with MM and is considered an emergency. Patients present with severe back pain, weakness of the lower extremities, and bladder or bowel incontinence. MRI should be performed immediately and treatment instituted with chemotherapy, radiotherapy, or neurosurgery to avoid permanent neurologic deficit.

SPEP detects a monoclonal protein in approximately 80% of patients with MM. The rate of detection increases to 90% with immunofixation and to more than 95% with serum FLC ratio. The distribution of types of monoclonal protein is as follows:

- IgG: 50% to 55%
- IgA: 20% to 25%
- Kappa or lambda light chain only: 15% to 20%
- IgD: 1% to 2%
- IgM 0.5% to 1%
- Biclonal: 1% to 2%
- Nonsecretory: 3% to 5%

A bone marrow aspirate and biopsy are key components to the diagnosis of MM. The percentage of involvement should be quantified from a core biopsy. Clonality is established by identifying light chain restriction by flow cytometry or immunohistochemistry.

DIAGNOSTIC CRITERIA FOR MULTIPLE MYELOMA ACCORDING TO THE REVISED INTERNATIONAL MYELOMA WORKING GROUP
Definition of Multiple Myeloma

Clonal bone marrow plasma cells greater than or equal to 10% OR biopsy-proven bone or soft tissue plasmacytoma, AND one or more of the following[31]:

- Hypercalcemia: serum calcium greater than 11 mg/dL
- Renal insufficiency: creatinine clearance less than 40 mL/min or serum creatinine greater than 2 mg/dL

- Anemia: hemoglobin less than 10 g/dL
- Bone lesions: osteolytic lesions on radiographs, CT, or PET/CT

The following represent an 80% risk of developing active MM within 2 years and should be considered active MM:

- Clonal bone marrow plasma cell involvement greater than or equal to 60%
- Serum FLC ratio greater than or equal to 100; kappa:lambda in kappa-restricted myeloma or lambda:kappa in lambda-restricted myeloma
- Greater than 1 focal lesion on MRI

Once the diagnosis of MM is made, the patients should undergo staging for prognostic purposes. The International Staging System (ISS) has become the preferred staging system given its simplicity.[32]

- ISS I: serum β-2-microglobulin less than 3.5 mg/L and serum albumin greater than 3.5 g/dL
- ISS II: neither stage I nor stage III
- ISS III: serum β-2-microglobulin greater than or equal to 5.5 mg/L

The median survival of MM patients with ISS stage I, II, and III is 62, 44, and 29 months, respectively.

The revised ISS (R-ISS) incorporates serum lactate dehydrogenase (LDH) and high-risk chromosomal abnormalities detected by fluorescence in situ hybridization (FISH).[33] The latter includes del(17p), t(4;14), and t(14;16).

- R-ISS stage I: ISS stage I AND normal serum LDH AND no high-risk FISH abnormalities
- R-ISS stage II: neither R-ISS stage I nor stage III
- R-ISS stage III: ISS stage III AND serum LDH above normal limits AND/OR detection of one of the high-risk FISH abnormalities.

The 5-year survival rates for R-ISS stages I, II, and III were 82%, 62%, and 40%, respectively.

Patient-related factors associated with worse prognosis include older age, poor performance status, higher serum creatinine and calcium, lower hemoglobin and platelet count, and higher bone marrow involvement. Also, non-IgG MM, circulating plasma cells, and abnormal FLC ratio have been associated with worse outcomes.

Before initiation of therapy, eligibility for autologous stem cell transplantation (ASCT) should be determined. Patients who are eligible for ASCT should not receive stem cell toxic drugs (eg, melphalan) as part of the induction treatment. The combination of the proteasome inhibitor bortezomib, the immunomodulator lenalidomide, and dexamethasone (RVD) is commonly used in ASCT-eligible and -ineligible patients with MM. RVD is associated with a response rate of 100% with a reasonable toxicity profile.[34] Lenalidomide needs adjustment for renal insufficiency. The combination of the alkylator cyclophosphamide, bortezomib, and dexamethasone has also shown efficacy with a response rate of 80% and does not need adjusted for renal dysfunction.[35] Other treatment options include but are not limited to bortezomib, thalidomide, and dexamethasone, bortezomib and dexamethasone, and lenalidomide and dexamethasone (RD). Bortezomib can be given weekly and subcutaneously to decrease risk of neurotoxicity. Patients on proteasome inhibitor therapy should receive prophylaxis against herpes zoster. In elderly patients, 2-drug combinations are safe and effective; however, lenalidomide and dexamethasone might need to be dose-reduced to minimize toxicity. In eligible patients, once induction therapy is completed, the standard approach is to proceed with high-dose chemotherapy followed by ASCT. ASCT-ineligible patients can receive regimens containing stem cell toxic agents, such as melphalan. The duration of induction varies depending on the regimen. Patients on melphalan or bortezomib-containing regimens continue therapy until a response plateau is reached (usually at 12–18 months). Patients on RD typically continue therapy until progression or unacceptable toxicity.

Response to therapy is assessed using serum monoclonal protein, immunofixation, serum FLC ratio, flow cytometry, and molecular studies.

INTERNATIONAL MYELOMA WORKING GROUP RESPONSE CRITERIA FOR MULTIPLE MYELOMA

- Molecular complete response: Stringent complete response AND no identifiable oligonucleotides on polymerase chain reaction[36]
- Immunophenotypic complete response: Stringent complete response AND no detectable aberrant clonal plasma cells by flow cytometry analysis of the bone marrow
- Stringent complete response: Complete response AND normal FLC ratio AND no clonal cells in the bone marrow by immunohistochemistry
- Complete response: No monoclonal protein in serum and urine by immunofixation AND no evidence of plasmacytoma AND bone marrow showing less than 5% plasma cells
- Very good partial response: monoclonal protein detectable by immunofixation but not electrophoresis or at least 90% reduction in serum monoclonal protein
- Partial response: At least 50% reduction in serum monoclonal protein AND at least 50% reduction in size of plasmacytomas
- Stable disease: Does not meet criteria for complete, very good partial or partial response, or progressive disease
- Progressive disease: At least 25% increase from lowest response value in serum or urine monoclonal protein, bone marrow plasma cell percentage, or difference in the serum FLC levels OR increase in size or new bone lesions or plasmacytomas

Almost all patients with MM who survive initial treatment will eventually experience relapse requiring therapy. Treatment options for relapsed disease include ASCT, use of the previous regimen, or a new regimen, including clinical trials. The novel proteasome inhibitors carfilzomib and ixazomib, the novel immunomodulatory drug pomalidomide, the histone deacetylase inhibitor panobinostat, and the monoclonal antibodies daratumumab (anti-CD38) and elotuzumab (anti-SMF7) have recently gained US Food and Drug Administration (FDA) approval for the treatment of patients with MM. Overall, the 5-year overall survival rate in patients with MM has increased from 40% before 2000 to higher than 60% after 2010, with larger survival benefits observed in patients older than 65 years.[37]

Smoldering Multiple Myeloma

Patients with smoldering MM meet all the criteria for active MM with exception of end-organ damage. The definition of smoldering MM includes serum monoclonal protein greater than or equal to 30 g/L OR urinary protein greater than or equal to 500 mg per 24 hours AND/OR clonal bone marrow plasma cells 10% to 60% AND absence of myeloma-defining events or amyloidosis. The rate of progression to active MM or AL amyloidosis occurs at a rate of 10% per year for the first 5 years, 3% per year for the next 5 years, and 1% to 2% per year for the following 10 years.[38] Three factors have been associated with progression from smoldering to active MM: abnormal serum FLC ratio, bone marrow plasma cells greater than or equal to 10%, and serum monoclonal protein greater than or equal to 3 g/dL. The rate of progression at 5 years was 25%, 51% and 76% for patients with 1, 2, or 3 risk factors, respectively.[38,39] After initial diagnosis, follow-up visit can span from every 3 to every 12 months depending on stability of the values. Similar to patients with MGUS, patients with smoldering MM have higher risk of fractures, thromboembolic disease, and secondary cancers. A group of patients with high-risk smoldering MM might benefit from early intervention with lenalidomide and dexamethasone.[40] However, additional studies are needed to standardize the treatment of patients with high-risk smoldering MM.

WALDENSTRÖM MACROGLOBULINEMIA

LPL/WM is a B-cell disorder characterized by the malignant accumulation of clonally related B cells, lymphoplasmacytic cells, and plasma cells in the bone marrow and other tissues.[41] LPL/WM is a rare disease with an incidence of 1000 new cases per year in the United States. The median age at diagnosis is 70 years, and less than 10% of patients are younger than 50 years.[42] More than 80% of patients are white, and about 20% are of Ashkenazi Jewish descent. About 20% of patients have a positive family history of hematologic malignancy in first-degree relatives.

The most common presenting symptoms in patients with LPL/WM are as follows:

- Fatigue/tiredness 40% to 50%, due to anemia
- Constitutional symptoms 25% to 30%
- Neurologic symptoms 20% to 25%, usually symmetric sensory neuropathy in lower extremities with evidence of demyelination in electromyography
- Symptoms of hyperviscosity 10% to 20%, such as nosebleeds, blurred vision, and headaches. A funduscopic examination should be performed in patients with typical symptoms, and if signs of hyperviscosity are seen (eg, increased tortuosity and sausaging of retinal vessels, retinal hemorrhages), plasmapheresis should be instituted urgently.
- Lymphadenopathy 10% to 15%
- Hepatosplenomegaly 10% to 15%

Other rare symptoms can be associated with cryoglobulinemia (vasculitic rash, non-healing ulcers in lower extremities), cold agglutinemia (hemolysis, hemoglobinuria), and amyloidosis. Renal involvement and bone lytic lesions in LPL/WM are rare.

The diagnosis of LPL/WM is made based on findings in the bone marrow biopsy, SPEP, and the clinical scenario. The following criteria must be met[43]:

- A serum IgM monoclonal protein of any size
- Involvement of the bone marrow by an intertrabecular infiltrate of any size of small lymphocytes, lymphoplasmacytoid forms, and plasma cells
- The lymphocytic cells typically express surface IgM, CD19, CD20, and CD22. The plasmacytic cells express CD38 and CD138.

More than 90% of patients with LPL/WM carry the recurrent MYD88 L265P gene mutation, which can help secure the diagnosis.[44] The MYD88 L265P mutation can be identified in about 50% of patients with IgM MGUS.

Initial evaluation of patients with LPL/WM should include the following:

- Laboratory studies: CBC, liver and kidney function, LDH, SPEP, and immunofixation, quantitative immunoglobulins, β-2-microglobulin, and serum FLC. In special cases, workup can include cryoglobulins, cold agglutinins, and von Willebrand disease screening

- Bone marrow aspiration and biopsy
- CT scans of the chest, abdomen, and pelvis with intravenous contrast
- Patients with neuropathy should undergo electromyograph (EMG) studies, and if demyelination is identified, then be tested for anti-myelin-associated glycoprotein antibodies.
- Amyloidosis should be evaluated by means of a fat pad biopsy stained with Congo red.

Approximately 25% to 35% of patients with LPL/WM do not meet criteria for initiation of therapy at diagnosis. Immediate treatment is not needed in all LPL/WM given its incurability and also prolonged survival. Criteria for initiation of therapy include the following[45]:

- Recurrent fever, night sweats, weight loss, and fatigue
- Hyperviscosity
- Symptomatic lymphadenopathy
- Symptomatic hepatomegaly and/or splenomegaly
- Symptomatic organomegaly and/or organ or tissue infiltration
- Peripheral neuropathy due to LPL/WM
- Hemoglobin less than or equal to 10 g/dL
- Platelet count less than $100 \times 10^9/L$
- Symptomatic cryoglobulinemia
- Symptomatic cold agglutinin anemia
- Autoimmune cytopenias
- Systemic amyloidosis

Primary therapy for LPL/WM should be reserved for patients with symptomatic disease. There is no clear advantage for early therapy. Patients who are eligible for ASCT should not receive stem cell toxic drugs. In patients with symptomatic hyperviscosity, plasmapheresis should be instituted urgently and followed by definitive therapy directed at LPL/WM. Most primary treatment regimens for LPL/WM are recommended based on single-arm prospective studies. The Bruton tyrosine kinase inhibitor ibrutinib is the only FDA-approved agent in the frontline and relapsed settings for patients with LPL/WM.[46] Commonly used regimens include alkylators (bendamustine or cyclophosphamide) or proteasome inhibitors (bortezomib or carfilzomib) in combination with the anti-CD20 monoclonal antibody rituximab.[47–49] Rituximab can also be used as a single agent. Rituximab should be used with caution in patients with LPL/WM with serum IgM levels greater than 4000 mg/dL as, in up to 40% of patients, rituximab therapy can be associated with an IgM flare that can be symptomatic. Such an IgM flare does not represent progression of disease. About 7% of LPL/WM patients exposed to rituximab can become intolerant to it, and ofatumumab can be used in such cases.[50]

Response to therapy is assessed using serum IgM levels, SPEP, and immunofixation, bone marrow biopsy, and CT scans.

INTERNATIONAL WORKING GROUP ON WALDENSTRÖM MACROGLOBULINEMIA RESPONSE CRITERIA

- Complete response: normal serum IgM level, disappearance of monoclonal protein on immunofixation, resolution of extramedullary disease, and resolution of signs and symptoms attributed to WM.[51]
- Very good partial response: At least 90% reduction in serum IgM, resolution of extramedullary disease, and resolution of signs and symptoms attributed to WM.
- Partial response: At least 50% but less than 90% decrease in serum IgM level AND at least 50% decrease in extramedullary disease.

- Minor response: At least 25% but less than 50% reduction in serum IgM level.
- Stable disease: Neither minor response or progressive disease.
- Progressive disease: Two measurements showing at least 25% increase in serum IgM level or progression of clinically significant cytopenias, extramedullary disease or constitutional symptoms, hyperviscosity, neuropathy, cryoglobuline-mia, or amyloidosis.

All patients with LPL/WM will eventually relapse after primary therapy. Treatment options for relapsed disease include the same regimen used for primary therapy, another frontline regimen, including clinical trials and, in exceptional cases, ASCT. Other agents used in the relapsed setting include thalidomide, lenalidomide, everoli-mus, fludarabine, cladribine, and chlorambucil.

A commonly used prognostic tool is the International Prognostic Scoring System for WM, which includes age greater than 65 years, hemoglobin less than or equal to 11.5 g/dL, platelet count less than or equal to 100×10^9/L, β-2-microglobulin greater than 3 mg/dL, and serum IgM greater than 7000 mg/dL. Patients are stratified in low-, intermediate-, and high-risk categories with 5-year survival rates of 87%, 68%, and 36%, respectively.[52] However, the patients included in such a study were not treated with novel regimens. High von Willebrand antigen level has been associated with a worse outcome.[53] Overall, the median survival on patients with LPL/WM has improved from 6 years in the 1990s to higher than 8 years in the 2000s.[42]

LIGHT CHAIN AMYLOIDOSIS

Light chain amyloidosis (AL amyloidosis) refers to the extracellular tissue deposition of monoclonal light chain fibrils. Patients can have AL amyloidosis alone or in association with other plasma cell disorders such as MGUS, MM, and LPL/WM. The incidence of AL amyloidosis is unknown. The median age at presentation is 64 years with men accounting for 70% of the cases.

The clinical presentation depends on the organs affected. Common organs affected include the following:

- Kidney (70%): asymptomatic proteinuria or nephrotic syndrome
- Heart (60%): restrictive cardiomyopathy or arrhythmias
- Nervous system, peripheral (20%) or autonomic (15%), characterized as numb-ness, paresthesias, carpal tunnel syndrome, orthostatic hypotension
- Gastrointestinal tract and liver: bleeding, gastroparesis, malabsorption, liver enzyme elevation
- Soft tissue: macroglossia, shoulder pad
- Skin: purpura, easy bruisability, subcutaneous nodules
- Bleeding: associated with factor X deficiency

Once the diagnosis is suspected, demonstration of amyloid fibrils should be pur-sued by biopsy of less invasive sites such as fat pad, rectal area, or bone marrow or, if negative, the affected organ. The diagnosis of AL amyloidosis requires all the following[31]:

- Presence of an amyloid-related systemic syndrome
- Positive staining by Congo red in any tissue
- Evidence the amyloid is light chain-related using spectrometry or electron microscopy
- Evidence of monoclonal plasma cell disorder

Initial evaluation of patients with AL amyloidosis should include the following:

- Laboratory studies: CBC, chemistries with liver and renal function, international normalized ratio, partial thromboplastin time, SPEP, and UPEP with immuno-fixation, serum FLC ratio, 24-hour urine protein, troponin, NT-proBNP, thyrotropin, and cortisol level. Factor X levels should be checked in special situations.
- Bone marrow aspirate and biopsy with Congo red staining
- Cardiac involvement should be evaluated with 12-lead electrocardiogram and echocardiogram. Cardiac MRI should be done in special situations
- Patients with neuropathy should undergo EMG studies
- Gastrointestinal involvement can be evaluated with stool guaiac studies, liver ul-trasound, and/or gastric-emptying studies

In patients eligible for ASCT, high-dose melphalan followed by ASCT can be used as initial therapy.[54] If delays in ASCT are expected, induction with bortezomib-based regimen is preferred. In patients who are ineligible for ASCT, which account for approximately 75% of the cases, melphalan or bortezomib-based regimens have shown efficacy.[55] In the relapsed setting, combination regimens with agents such as melphalan, cyclophosphamide, bendamustine, bortezomib, thalidomide, lenalido-mide, and pomalidomide have been investigated in prospective studies.[56–60]

Response to treatment can be assessed with SPEP, UPEP, serum and urine immu-nofixation, serum FLC levels, and markers specific to the organs affected.

ROUNDTABLE ON CLINICAL RESEARCH IN LIGHT-CHAIN AMYLOIDOSIS RESPONSE CRITERIA
Hematologic Response

- Complete response: Normalization of FLC levels and ratio, negative urine, and serum immunofixation[61]
- Very good partial response: Reduction in the difference between involved and uninvolved FLC (dFLC) to less than 40 mg/L
- Partial response: A greater than 50% reduction in the dFLC
- No response: Less than partial response
- Progression: FLC increase of 50% to greater than 100 mg/L; if patient achieved complete remission, any detectable monoclonal protein, or abnormal FLC ratio. If patient achieved partial response, 50% increase in monoclonal protein to greater than 0.5 g/dL or 50% increase in urine monoclonal protein to greater than 200 mg/d

Specific criteria for organ response and progression have been published.

The prognosis of AL amyloidosis varies greatly. Poor survival has been consistently reported in patients with cardiac or liver failure and is typically measured in a few months.[62] On the other hand, patients with limited organ disease can have survival times more than 5 years. Patients with concurrent AL amyloidosis and myeloma tend to have a worse prognosis than AL amyloidosis alone.[63] Other adverse prognostic fac-tors are elevated NT-proBNP, elevated troponin, elevated uric acid, and dFLC.

POLYNEUROPATHY, ORGANOMEGALY, ENDOCRINOPATHY, MONOCLONAL PROTEIN, AND SKIN CHANGES SYNDROME

POEMS syndrome is a rare disorder that affects patients in the fifth to sixth decade of life. The clinical manifestations are highly variable. According to the IMWG, the diagnosis of POEMS syndrome is made by the presence of 2 mandatory criteria in addition to one major and one minor criterion.[31]

Mandatory Criteria

- Peripheral neuropathy, clinically sensorimotor with evidence of axonal and demyelinating damage in EMG studies
- Monoclonal plasma cell disorder, characterized by serum or urine monoclonal protein, typically lambda restricted. Bone marrow biopsy might be unrevealing.

Major Criteria

- Osteosclerotic bone lesions, which can be detected by plain radiographs or CT scans. Biopsy of these lesions show light chain–restricted plasma cells.
- Increased vascular endothelial growth factor (VEGF) levels, of at least 3 to 4 times the upper limit of normal
- Castleman disease, observed in lymph node biopsy

Minor Criteria

- Endocrine abnormalities, such as hypogonadism, high follicle stimulating hormone levels, adrenal insufficiency, hypothyroidism, and diabetes mellitus
- Skin changes, such as hyperpigmentation, hemangiomas, or hypertrichosis
- Organomegaly, such as hepatomegaly, splenomegaly, or lymphadenopathy
- Extravascular volume overload, such as ascites, peripheral edema, or pleural effusion
- Hematologic abnormalities, such as leukocytosis, thrombocytosis, or polycythemia
- Papilledema

There is no standard treatment for POEMS syndrome. Radiotherapy can be used for the management of localized disease (eg, 1–3 isolated bone lesions). For more widespread disease, similar treatment to MM is recommended. In young patients with widespread disease or severe neuropathy, high-dose chemotherapy followed by ASCT can be considered. Formal response criteria have not been published. However, CBC, serum monoclonal protein, SPEP and immunofixation, VEGF levels, and PET/CT can be used for response assessment. The median survival is longer than patients with myeloma at about 14 years.[64] Neuropathy is typically progressive, reaching disability in most cases. Most common causes of death are infections and cardiorespiratory failure.

SUMMARY

Plasma cell disorders are benign, premalignant, and malignant processes characterized by the presence of a monoclonal protein in the serum or urine. Clinically and biologically, these disorders are heterogeneous. However, there have been substantial advances in the understanding of the biology of these diseases that have prompted improvements in treatment, which are translating into better survival rates and quality of life. Additional research should focus on improving the efficacy as well as the short- and long-term toxicity profile of our interventions.

REFERENCES

1. Axelsson U. A 20-year follow-up study of 64 subjects with M-components. Acta Med Scand 1986;219(5):519–22.

2. Kyle RA, Finkelstein S, Elveback LR, et al. Incidence of monoclonal proteins in a Minnesota community with a cluster of multiple myeloma. Blood 1972;40(5): 719–24.

3. Saleun JP, Vicariot M, Deroff P, et al. Monoclonal gammopathies in the adult population of Finistere, France. J Clin Pathol 1982;35(1):63–8.

4. Kyle RA, Therneau TM, Rajkumar SV, et al. Prevalence of monoclonal gammopathy of undetermined significance. N Engl J Med 2006;354(13):1362–9.

5. Landgren O, Gridley G, Turesson I, et al. Risk of monoclonal gammopathy of undetermined significance (MGUS) and subsequent multiple myeloma among African American and white veterans in the United States. Blood 2006;107(3):904–6.

6. Iwanaga M, Tagawa M, Tsukasaki K, et al. Prevalence of monoclonal gammopathy of undetermined significance: study of 52,802 persons in Nagasaki City, Japan. Mayo Clin Proc 2007;82(12):1474–9.

7. Ruiz-Delgado GJ, Gomez Rangel JD. Monoclonal gammopathy of undetermined significance (MGUS) in Mexican mestizos: one institution's experience. Gac Med Mex 2004;140(4):375–9 [in Spanish].

8. Landgren O, Kristinsson SY, Goldin LR, et al. Risk of plasma cell and lymphoproliferative disorders among 14621 first-degree relatives of 4458 patients with monoclonal gammopathy of undetermined significance in Sweden. Blood 2009; 114(4):791–5.

9. Vachon CM, Kyle RA, Therneau TM, et al. Increased risk of monoclonal gammopathy in first-degree relatives of patients with multiple myeloma or monoclonal gammopathy of undetermined significance. Blood 2009;114(4):785–90.

10. Therneau TM, Kyle RA, Melton LJ 3rd, et al. Incidence of monoclonal gammopathy of undetermined significance and estimation of duration before first clinical recognition. Mayo Clin Proc 2012;87(11):1071–9.

11. Kyle RA, Therneau TM, Rajkumar SV, et al. A long-term study of prognosis in monoclonal gammopathy of undetermined significance. N Engl J Med 2002; 346(8):564–9.

12. Rajkumar SV, Kyle RA, Buadi FK. Advances in the diagnosis, classification, risk stratification, and management of monoclonal gammopathy of undetermined significance: implications for recategorizing disease entities in the presence of evolving scientific evidence. Mayo Clin Proc 2010;85(10):945–8.

13. Kyle RA, Therneau TM, Rajkumar SV, et al. Long-term follow-up of IgM monoclonal gammopathy of undetermined significance. Blood 2003;102(10):3759–64.

14. Dispenzieri A, Katzmann JA, Kyle RA, et al. Prevalence and risk of progression of light-chain monoclonal gammopathy of undetermined significance: a retrospective population-based cohort study. Lancet 2010;375(9727):1721–8.

15. Rajkumar SV, Kyle RA, Therneau TM, et al. Serum free light chain ratio is an independent risk factor for progression in monoclonal gammopathy of undetermined significance. Blood 2005;106(3):812–7.

16. Turesson I, Kovalchik SA, Pfeiffer RM, et al. Monoclonal gammopathy of undetermined significance and risk of lymphoid and myeloid malignancies: 728 cases followed up to 30 years in Sweden. Blood 2014;123(3):338–45.

17. Kyle RA, Durie BG, Rajkumar SV, et al. Monoclonal gammopathy of undetermined significance (MGUS) and smoldering (asymptomatic) multiple myeloma: IMWG consensus perspectives risk factors for progression and guidelines for monitoring and management. Leukemia 2010;24(6):1121–7.

18. Varettoni M, Corso A, Cocito F, et al. Changing pattern of presentation in monoclonal gammopathy of undetermined significance: a single-center experience with 1400 patients. Medicine (Baltimore) 2010;89(4):211–6.

19. Kristinsson SY, Fears TR, Gridley G, et al. Deep vein thrombosis after monoclonal gammopathy of undetermined significance and multiple myeloma. Blood 2008; 112(9):3582–6.

20. Kristinsson SY, Pfeiffer RM, Bjorkholm M, et al. Arterial and venous thrombosis in monoclonal gammopathy of undetermined significance and multiple myeloma: a population-based study. Blood 2010;115(24):4991–8.

21. Kristinsson SY, Tang M, Pfeiffer RM, et al. Monoclonal gammopathy of undetermined significance and risk of skeletal fractures: a population-based study. Blood 2010;116(15):2651–5.

22. Mailankody S, Pfeiffer RM, Kristinsson SY, et al. Risk of acute myeloid leukemia and myelodysplastic syndromes after multiple myeloma and its precursor disease (MGUS). Blood 2011;118(15):4086–92.

23. Roeker LE, Larson DR, Kyle RA, et al. Risk of acute leukemia and myelodysplastic syndromes in patients with monoclonal gammopathy of undetermined significance (MGUS): a population-based study of 17 315 patients. Leukemia 2013; 27(6):1391–3.

24. Za T, De Stefano V, Rossi E, et al. Arterial and venous thrombosis in patients with monoclonal gammopathy of undetermined significance: incidence and risk factors in a cohort of 1491 patients. Br J Haematol 2013;160(5):673–9.

25. Kyle RA, Therneau TM, Rajkumar SV, et al. Incidence of multiple myeloma in Olmsted County, Minnesota: trend over 6 decades. Cancer 2004;101(11): 2667–74.

26. Siegel RL, Miller KD, Jemal A. Cancer statistics, 2016. CA Cancer J Clin 2016; 66(1):7–30.

27. Kyle RA, Gertz MA, Witzig TE, et al. Review of 1027 patients with newly diagnosed multiple myeloma. Mayo Clin Proc 2003;78(1):21–33.

28. Huang SY, Yao M, Tang JL, et al. Epidemiology of multiple myeloma in Taiwan: increasing incidence for the past 25 years and higher prevalence of extramedullary myeloma in patients younger than 55 years. Cancer 2007;110(4):896–905.

29. Waxman AJ, Mink PJ, Devesa SS, et al. Racial disparities in incidence and outcome in multiple myeloma: a population-based study. Blood 2010;116(25): 5501–6.

30. Lynch HT, Sanger WG, Pirruccello S, et al. Familial multiple myeloma: a family study and review of the literature. J Natl Cancer Inst 2001;93(19):1479–83.

31. Rajkumar SV, Dimopoulos MA, Palumbo A, et al. International myeloma working group updated criteria for the diagnosis of multiple myeloma. Lancet Oncol 2014;15(12):e538–48.

32. Greipp PR, San Miguel J, Durie BG, et al. International staging system for multiple myeloma. J Clin Oncol 2005;23(15):3412–20.

33. Palumbo A, Avet-Loiseau H, Oliva S, et al. Revised international staging system for multiple myeloma: a report from international myeloma working group. J Clin Oncol 2015;33(26):2863–9.

34. Richardson PG, Weller E, Lonial S, et al. Lenalidomide, bortezomib, and dexamethasone combination therapy in patients with newly diagnosed multiple myeloma. Blood 2010;116(5):679–86.

35. Kumar S, Flinn I, Richardson PG, et al. Randomized, multicenter, phase 2 study (EVOLUTION) of combinations of bortezomib, dexamethasone, cyclophosphamide, and lenalidomide in previously untreated multiple myeloma. Blood 2012; 119(19):4375–82.

36. Kyle RA, Rajkumar SV. Criteria for diagnosis, staging, risk stratification and response assessment of multiple myeloma. Leukemia 2009;23(1):3–9.

37. Kumar SK, Dispenzieri A, Lacy MQ, et al. Continued improvement in survival in multiple myeloma: changes in early mortality and outcomes in older patients. Leukemia 2014;28(5):1122–8.

38. Kyle RA, Remstein ED, Therneau TM, et al. Clinical course and prognosis of smoldering (asymptomatic) multiple myeloma. N Engl J Med 2007;356(25):2582–90.

39. Dispenzieri A, Kyle RA, Katzmann JA, et al. Immunoglobulin free light chain ratio is an independent risk factor for progression of smoldering (asymptomatic) multiple myeloma. Blood 2008;111(2):785–9.

40. Mateos MV, Hernandez MT, Giraldo P, et al. Lenalidomide plus dexamethasone for high-risk smoldering multiple myeloma. N Engl J Med 2013;369(5):438–47.

41. Swerdlow SH, Berger F, Pileri SA, et al. Lymphoplasmacytic lymphoma. In: Swerdlow SH, Campo E, Harris NL, et al, editors. WHO classification of tumours of haematopoietic and lymphoid tissues. Lyon (France): IARC; 2008. p. 194–5.

42. Castillo JJ, Olszewski AJ, Kanan S, et al. Overall survival and competing risks of death in patients with Waldenstrom macroglobulinaemia: an analysis of the surveillance, epidemiology and end results database. Br J Haematol 2015;169(1): 81–9.

43. Owen RG, Treon SP, Al-Katib A, et al. Clinicopathological definition of Waldenstrom's macroglobulinemia: consensus panel recommendations from the second international workshop on Waldenstrom's macroglobulinemia. Semin Oncol 2003; 30(2):110–5.

44. Treon SP, Xu L, Yang G, et al. MYD88 L265P somatic mutation in Waldenstrom's macroglobulinemia. N Engl J Med 2012;367(9):826–33.

45. Kyle RA, Treon SP, Alexanian R, et al. Prognostic markers and criteria to initiate therapy in Waldenstrom's macroglobulinemia: consensus panel recommendations from the second international workshop on Waldenstrom's macroglobulinemia. Semin Oncol 2003;30(2):116–20.

46. Treon SP, Tripsas CK, Meid K, et al. Ibrutinib in previously treated Waldenstrom's macroglobulinemia. N Engl J Med 2015;372(15):1430–40.

47. Rummel MJ, Niederle N, Maschmeyer G, et al. Bendamustine plus rituximab versus CHOP plus rituximab as first-line treatment for patients with indolent and mantle-cell lymphomas: an open-label, multicentre, randomised, phase 3 non-inferiority trial. Lancet 2013;381(9873):1203–10.

48. Treon SP, Ioakimidis L, Soumerai JD, et al. Primary therapy of Waldenstrom macroglobulinemia with bortezomib, dexamethasone, and rituximab: WMCTG clinical trial 05-180. J Clin Oncol 2009;27(23):3830–5.

49. Treon SP, Tripsas CK, Meid K, et al. Carfilzomib, rituximab, and dexamethasone (CaRD) treatment offers a neuropathy-sparing approach for treating Waldenstrom's macroglobulinemia. Blood 2014;124(4):503–10.

50. Castillo JJ, Kanan S, Meid K, et al. Rituximab intolerance in patients with Waldenstrom macroglobulinaemia. Br J Haematol 2016;174(4):645–8.

51. Owen RG, Kyle RA, Stone MJ, et al. Response assessment in Waldenstrom macroglobulinaemia: update from the VIth International Workshop. Br J Haematol 2013;160(2):171–6.

52. Morel P, Duhamel A, Gobbi P, et al. International prognostic scoring system for Waldenstrom macroglobulinemia. Blood 2009;113(18):4163–70.

53. Hivert B, Caron C, Petit S, et al. Clinical and prognostic implications of low or high level of von Willebrand factor in patients with Waldenstrom macroglobulinemia. Blood 2012;120(16):3214–21.

54. Dispenzieri A, Lacy MQ, Kyle RA, et al. Eligibility for hematopoietic stem-cell transplantation for primary systemic amyloidosis is a favorable prognostic factor for survival. J Clin Oncol 2001;19(14):3350–6.
55. Venner CP, Lane T, Foard D, et al. Cyclophosphamide, bortezomib, and dexamethasone therapy in AL amyloidosis is associated with high clonal response rates and prolonged progression-free survival. Blood 2012;119(19):4387–90.
56. Dispenzieri A, Buadi F, Laumann K, et al. Activity of pomalidomide in patients with immunoglobulin light-chain amyloidosis. Blood 2012;119(23):5397–404.
57. Moreau P, Jaccard A, Benboubker L, et al. Lenalidomide in combination with melphalan and dexamethasone in patients with newly diagnosed AL amyloidosis: a multicenter phase 1/2 dose-escalation study. Blood 2010;116(23):4777–82.
58. Palladini G, Perfetti V, Perlini S, et al. The combination of thalidomide and intermediate-dose dexamethasone is an effective but toxic treatment for patients with primary amyloidosis (AL). Blood 2005;105(7):2949–51.
59. Reece DE, Hegenbart U, Sanchorawala V, et al. Efficacy and safety of once-weekly and twice-weekly bortezomib in patients with relapsed systemic AL amyloidosis: results of a phase 1/2 study. Blood 2011;118(4):865–73.
60. Sanchorawala V, Wright DG, Rosenzweig M, et al. Lenalidomide and dexamethasone in the treatment of AL amyloidosis: results of a phase 2 trial. Blood 2007; 109(2):492–6.
61. Palladini G, Dispenzieri A, Gertz MA, et al. New criteria for response to treatment in immunoglobulin light chain amyloidosis based on free light chain measurement and cardiac biomarkers: impact on survival outcomes. J Clin Oncol 2012;30(36): 4541–9.
62. Dispenzieri A, Seenithamby K, Lacy MQ, et al. Patients with immunoglobulin light chain amyloidosis undergoing autologous stem cell transplantation have superior outcomes compared with patients with multiple myeloma: a retrospective review from a tertiary referral center. Bone Marrow Transplant 2013;48(10):1302–7.
63. Pardanani A, Witzig TE, Schroeder G, et al. Circulating peripheral blood plasma cells as a prognostic indicator in patients with primary systemic amyloidosis. Blood 2003;101(3):827–30.
64. Dispenzieri A, Kyle RA, Lacy MQ, et al. POEMS syndrome: definitions and long-term outcome. Blood 2003;101(7):2496–506.

Basics of Hematopoietic Cell Transplantation for Primary Care Physicians and Internists

Shahrukh Khurshid Hashmi, MD, MPH*

KEYWORDS

- Bone marrow transplant • Stem cell transplant • Graft-versus-host disease
- Engraftment

KEY POINTS

- Hematopoietic cell transplant (HCT) activity is increasing worldwide.
- Longitudinal care for transplant survivors is frequently provided by primary care providers and internists.
- Transplant survivors can develop unique long-term complications due to chemotherapy and/or radiation exposure that primary care physicians and internists need to be aware of.

BASICS OF HEMATOPOIETIC CELL TRANSPLANTATION FOR PRIMARY CARE PHYSICIANS AND INTERNISTS

The field of HCT began more than 50 years ago when Dr Don Thomas started to perform bone marrow transplantation for cancers.[1] Fast forward half a century, more than 60,000 HCTs are performed worldwide annually to treat a variety of malignant and nonmalignant conditions. Although HCT is complicated and risky, a majority of the HCT recipients are surviving for many years post-transplant and are seen by nontransplant physicians, including hematologists, oncologists, internists, pediatricians, hospitalists, and primary care physicians for care delivery. There are few transplant centers given this is a specialized field; therefore, most patients travel for the receipt of HCT to a large medical institution and, once the required 1-month to 3-month stay in the vicinity of the transplant center is done, they return home. Hence, the longitudinal long-term care of HCT recipients is frequently dictated by primary care providers. The complications of this procedure are unique; thus, it requires an individualized care delivery plan to each patient. This article presents the basics of

This author has nothing to disclose.
Mayo Clinic, Rochester, MN 55901, USA
* Mayo Clinic, 200 First Street Southwest, Rochester, MN 55905.
E-mail address: hashmi.shahrukh@mayo.edu

transplantation, HCT types/stem cell sources, mobilization and conditioning procedures, indications for HCT, conditioning regimens, engraftment, graft-versus-host-disease, and lastly survivorship issues.

BASICS OF HEMATOPOIETIC CELL TRANSPLANTATION — TERMINOLOGY

The term, bone marrow transplantation, lexicographically is a misnomer. When this procedure started, donors were taken to an operating room, and from both the iliac crests, multiple bone marrow biopsies were obtained to get a sufficient amount of marrow. Over time with better recognition of hematopoietic stem cells and availability of mobilizing agents, HCTs have been facilitated by using stem cells obtained from a donor's blood. A majority (>70%) of the adult HCTs in the United States currently use peripheral blood stem cells (PBSCs) from donors; thus, both the terms, *stem cell transplantation* and *bone marrow transplantation*, colloquially used, constitute HCT.

TYPES OF HEMATOPOIETIC CELL TRANSPLANTATION AND DONOR STEM CELL SOURCES

The 3 types of HCT are syngeneic, autologous, and allogeneic (**Table 1**). Grafts or stem cells (or bone marrow) for syngeneic, autologous, and allogeneic HCTs are obtained from identical twins, self, or another nonidentical human donor, respectively. No xenografts (transplantation from one species to another species) are used in the field of HCT currently.

Approximately half of HCTs globally are autologous HCT. In the United States, because multiple myeloma and lymphomas are common, a majority of the HCTs are autologous HCT.[2] In autologous HCT, stem cells from recipients are obtained usually after their cancer goes into remission. The stem cells are then frozen and can be used any time for HCT.

For allogeneic HCT, a donor is selected based on many factors, most important of which is HLA matching at the allele level (HLA-A, HLA-B, HLA-C, HLA-DR, or HLA-DQ). Other factors that play a role in donor selection include ABO blood group match for donor/recipient [D/R], cytomegalovirus D/R, weight D/R, and age of the donor (younger donors are preferred).

A full match consists of allele-level matching at the 5 HLA antigens (therefore a 10/10 match!). Hence, a 9/10 allele match is considered a partially matched (mismatched) donor. In general, the 3 main donor sources for allogeneic HCT include (1) related donor, (2) unrelated donor, and (3) cord blood stem cells (obtained from an umbilical cord during childbirth).

Table 1 Types of hematopoietic cell transplantations			
Type	Source	Graft vs Tumor Effect	Comments
Syngeneic	From identical twin	None	Rarely used due to poor availability
Autologous	One's own stem cells	None	Mainly used for myelomas and lymphomas
Allogeneic	From another human	Yes	Can be obtained from related donors, unrelated donor or from the umbilical cord blood

1. Related donors: there is a 25% chance that a biologic sibling is a full match. If half matches (haploidentical) are considered, however, then there is a much greater likelihood of finding a match within family members for example, parents, children, and siblings. Testing for cousins and other relatives is low yield and therefore not encouraged.
b. Unrelated donors: currently, the world registry consists of 27 million volunteer donors,[2] and the chances of finding a full match within that registry is highly dependent on the race of an individual. White patients have a greater than 80% probability of finding a match in the world registry whereas Africans have less than 30% probability of finding a full match.[3] This is mainly due to the fact that most registrants in the world registry are white.
c. Cord blood units: more than 0.6 million units of frozen umbilical cord blood are available for HCTs and do not require a full match for a successful outcome.

MOBILIZATION AND CONDITIONING

Mobilization of stem cells is a procedure that is commonly done both in autologous HCT and allogeneic HCT to obtain PBSCs. Usually cytokines (eg, granulocyte-colony stimulating factor) are given for 3 to 5 days and then a donor (could be autologous or allogeneic) undergoes apheresis to collect a sufficient number of PBSCs. The minimum required dosage to ensure engraftment for a majority of the patients is greater than or equal to 2 million/kg CD34$^+$ (PBSC); however, most transplant centers target a higher dose for a single HCT (usually >3 million/kg CD34$^+$ cells) for better engraftment. Increasingly, a CXCR4 antagonist, plerixafor, is used for mobilization either alone or along with cytokines.

The preparative or conditioning regimen refers to the chemotherapy (or chemoradiation) administered just before the infusion of stem cells. Not infrequently this terminology is confusing to patients because it could be mistaken for another cycle of chemotherapy. Although this is chemotherapy, it is distinct from chemotherapy cycles in its purpose, constituents, and properties and SHOULD NEVER be administered outside the field of HCT because the dose of chemotherapy can be fatal unless stem cells are infused afterward. A conditioning regimen should be sufficient to cause myeloablation as well as immunoablation (the latter is necessary to minimize the risk of graft rejection).

There are 3 types of conditioning regimens: (1) myeloablative (MA), (2) reduced intensity conditioning (RIC), and (3) non-MA (NMA). By definition all autologous HCTs receive MA regimens and the distinction of the intensity of regimens is applicable to allogeneic HCT.

1. MA regimens: these regimens provide extremely high doses of chemotherapy with or without radiation therapy to a patient to cause myeloablation, immunoablation, and eradication of the disease. Typical examples are busulfan + cyclophosphamide and cyclophosphamide + total body irradiation (TBI). MA regimens are also known as full-intensity regimens. The dose of TBI is MA regimens is usually greater than 10 Gy.
2. NMA regimens: these regimens provide sufficient immunoablation for a successful engraftment but do not cause myeloablation. These regimens, when used in malignancies, use graft-versus-tumor effect to combat malignancies. A classic NMA regimen developed in Seattle uses only 2 Gy of TBI. Sometimes, the term, *mini-transplant*, is used for these regimens because they are less toxic than both MA and RIC regimens, notwithstanding that the complications of this type of conditioning can be severe. HCT experts recommend avoiding the term, minitransplant, because it can be misleading.

3. Reduced intensity regimens: all regimens that do not fit into NMA or MA are known as RIC, which are intermediate intensity.

Generally, RIC and NMA are more the frequently used regimens for elderly and unfit patients requiring HCT. The crude methods of assessing baseline health in HCT, like Karnofsky Performance Scale status, are not helpful in deciding whether a patient would be an appropriate candidate for a particular transplant regimen (or even for decision making to go ahead with a transplant or not). The gold standard for pretransplant assessment of health status of any patient is a validated tool called Hematopoietic Cell Transplantation Comorbidity Index, which assesses 17 different categories of organ dysfunction.[4]

INDICATIONS FOR TRANSPLANT

The indications for HCT are continuously expanding as the procedure becomes safer and logistically easier. Recently, the American Society of Blood and Marrow Transplantation (ASBMT) published guidelines with respect to the indications for both autologous HCT and allogeneic HCT.[5] In the United States, most common indication for allogeneic HCT is leukemia, whereas multiple myeloma is the most common indication for autologous transplantation. The common indications for HCT are discussed.

1. Allogeneic HCT
   a. Hematologic malignancies, for example, acute and chronic leukemias (acute myeloid leukemia [AML], acute lymphoid leukemia, chronic myeloid leukemia, and chronic lymphoid leukemia), myelodysplastic syndrome [MDSs], lymphomas (both Hodgkin and non-Hodgkin), multiple myeloma, and myeloproliferative neoplasms (eg, myelofibrosis and systemic mastocytosis)
   b. Inherited metabolic disorders — for example, mucopolysaccharidosis, adrenoleukodystrophy, metachromatic leukodystrophy, osteopetrosis, and others
   c. Inherited immune disorders, for example, severe combined immunodeficiency, Wiskott-Aldrich syndrome, GATA2 mutations (if causing clonal hematologic disorders), and others
   d. Inherited hemoglobinopathies, for example, sickle cell disease, β-thalassemia, and others
   e. Marrow failure states — severe aplastic anemia, Fanconi anemia, and others
   f. Allogeneic HCT in acquired HIV is considered experimental and currently is performed only if there is an associated hematologic disorder.
2. Autologous HCT
   a. Multiple myeloma
   b. Non-Hodgkin lymphoma
   c. Hodgkin lymphoma
   d. Autoimmune diseases (advanced scleroderma and multiple sclerosis): this is still considered experimental in the United States.
   e. Germ cell tumors
   f. Neuroblastoma

It is important to refer patients early in the disease course to a transplant center to get plugged in for an immediate or future HCT. Because the HLA typing and matching process may take upwards of 2 weeks and getting stem cells from a donor may take up to another 4 weeks, it is reasonable to get an HCT expert consult at the time of diagnosis of a high-risk malignancy, for example, a newly diagnosed AML with monosomy 7.

ENGRAFTMENT

Engraftment is the process whereby the donor stem cells begin to produce new blood components within the recipient's bone marrow niche. In practice, engraftment is said to have occurred when the absolute neutrophil count consistently exceeds $0.5 \times (10)^9$/L for 3 days in a row (without growth factor support). Platelet engraftment generally follows and is defined according to institutional standards. The red cell series do not affect the engraftment. The patient is supported with blood products until engraftment occurs; however, in some cases of NMA conditioned HCT, minimal or no transfusion support is needed. Engraftment typically occurs between day +12 and day +25 and is usually earlier when PBSCs are used in comparison to bone marrow. Graft failure in the current era of allele-level high-resolution matching is rare and occurs in less than 5% of the allogeneic HCTs. It is extremely rare to encounter a graft failure postautologous HCT.

Although engraftment is seen in a majority of cases, the reconstitution of T-cell and B-cell immunity can take up to a year or longer, so extreme caution to alleviate the risk of infections should be exercised. HCT recipients who are not on heavy doses of immunosuppression require reimmunization of essential vaccines at 6 to 12 months post-HCT.

GRAFT-VERSUS-HOST DISEASE

When the new immune system in a recipient of an allogeneic transplant attacks the recipient, the condition is called GVHD. For GVHD to occur, the Billingham criteria should be met:

1. An immunocompetent graft is administered, with viable and functional immune cells.
2. The recipient is immunologically different from the donor — histoincompatible.
3. The recipient is immunocompromised and, therefore, cannot destroy or inactivate the transplanted cells.

The pathophysiology of acute GVHD is still under investigation in human models, although canine and murine models have indicated that the T lymphocytes present in the allograft attack the tissues of the transplant recipient after perceiving host tissues as foreign. The T cells produce an excess of cytokines, including tumor necrosis factor α and interferon-γ, besides many other factors.[6] A wide range of host antigens can initiate GVHD; among them, HLA is the most common. Recently many minor antigens and other factors have been identified as playing a role in acute GVHD pathophysiology. Antigens/proteins that have been recently implicated in GVHD pathogenesis and are currently being evaluated in clinical trials include noninherited maternal antigens, KIR, and HLA-DPB1 variants (especially rs9277534 allele variant).[7]

The acute GVHD can be prevented by using a T-cell deplete (TCD) graft, which may require ex vivo or in vivo T cell depletion. Antithymocyte globulin and alemtuzumab are common methods used for TCD grafting in allogeneic HCT. For ex vivo TCD, the CliniMACS CD34 Reagent System can selectively collect hematopoietic stem cells from donor apheresis while passively depleting T cells. Recently, a large phase III randomized study has indicated significant benefit in reduction of GVHD when antithymocyte globulin was used (compared with placebo) with standard conditioning, without a compromise on overall survival.

The balance of donor cytotoxic or conventional T cells CD3$^+$/CD8$^+$ to helper or regulatory T cells is critical in transplants for hematologic malignancies. Although conventional T cells are undesirable as effector cells of GVHD, they are valuable for engraftment because they prevent the recipient's residual immune system from rejecting the bone marrow graft (host-versus-graft). In addition, donor T cells have proved to have a valuable graft-versus-tumor effect. A great deal of current research on HCT involves attempts to separate the undesirable GVHD aspects of T-cell physiology from the desirable graft-versus-tumor effect, a concept still considered the holy grail of transplantation.

Acute GVHD typically presents with involvement of 3 organ systems: liver, gastrointestinal (GI) tract, and the skin. Liver manifestation is usually a cholestasis picture but can present with severe transaminitis too. GI tract symptoms commonly include diarrhea and nausea/vomiting. Skin rashes classically present as sunburns, but commonly a variety of presentations are seen in practice ranging from a maculopapular rash to desquamative erythroderma.

Chronic GVHD is distinct with both B cells and T cells involved in pathogenesis; it involves almost all organ systems. Not infrequently, the clinical manifestations resemble classic autoimmune diseases, for example, Sjögren syndrome, scleroderma, and so forth. The initial treatment of both acute and chronic GVHD consists of high-dose corticosteroids. Approximately half of patients suffer from steroid refractory GVHD, which causes substantial morbidity and mortality, with less than 80% patients surviving long term. No Food and Drug Administration–approved therapies exist because none of the drug therapies has proved beneficial. Because there is no standard approach to second-line therapies, a discussion of pros and cons of various common agents used for treatment of GVHD is beyond the scope of this article. It is recommended that every steroid refractory GVHD patient be transferred to the original transplant center for complete evaluation and management.

HEMATOPOIETIC CELL TRANSPLANTATION SURVIVORSHIP ISSUES

Most transplant centers mandate that allogeneic HCT recipients stay in the geographic vicinity of the transplant center for at least 100 days post-transplant because many complications occur within months of transplant, including infections, organ failure, GVHD, and psychological issues. After that time period, most patients who are doing well travel back to their respective home towns and are cared for by their primary hematologists/oncologists and primary care providers. Some transplant centers mandate that HCT survivors return to their centers yearly, but published data have indicated vulnerabilities in the transition of care of these survivors and many are lost in transition.

HCT can lead to many unique complications that require a specified surveillance plan and considerable expertise. GVHD is a unique condition that can affect organ functions at any time post-HCT. Its management is difficult and best handled by GVHD experts. Additionally, the chemotherapy or radiation given at the time of transplant can lead to conditions associated with accelerated aging and include second cancers (significantly higher risk of skin/oral cavity and other solid cancers), therapy-related myeloid neoplasms (AML and MDS), premature atherosclerosis (including coronary artery disease), endocrine abnormalities, and infertility. Childhood cancer survivor studies indicate that compared with healthy siblings, the recipients of allogeneic HCT had significantly elevated risk of these conditions years after HCT.[8] These complications are known as late effects in the HCT literature.

Most developed countries have devised national guidelines for screening and prevention of complications of common chronic medical illnesses from cancer screening to deafness screening. The United States Preventive Services Task Force is an independent panel of experts in primary care and prevention that systematically reviews evidence of effectiveness and develops recommendations for clinical preventive services. These recommendations (or any other national recommendations) do not apply to HCT survivors because they are targeted toward the general population. The Center for International Blood and Marrow Transplant Research, the European Group for Blood and Marrow Transplantation, and the ASBMT convened a group of experts and provided consensus recommendations for screening and preventive practices for HCT survivors, which are published on-line at their respective Web sites.[9] Generally, it is strongly recommended that all HCT survivors visit their respective transplant centers annually even if they are completely asymptomatic. There are different types of survivorship clinics (or long-term follow-up [LTFU] clinics) present in different institutions and referral should be made to the closest HCT LTFU program in the absence of an established LTFU clinic at the original transplant center. **Table 2** depicts the various types of HCT survivorship programs.[10]

Table 2
Hematopoietic stem cell transplant survivor clinic models

Clinic Model	Advantages	Disadvantages
Cancer survivorship integrated model (no strictly defined interval of post-HSCT duration for inclusion)	Initiation is relatively easy given the already existent cancer survivorship clinic May have extensive collaborations with various specialties for both cancer and HSCT care	Dedicated GVHD experts may not be available to evaluate all HSCT patients More intense utilization of resources and time for clinical and supportive services may not be affordable
	Excellent systems in place for systems-based practice with community clinicians	Lack of knowledge of late effects of HSCT survivors of nonmalignant diseases, for example, hemoglobinopathies, bone marrow failure syndromes
Chronic GVHD and survivorship LTFU (may start at 6 mo to 2 y after HSCT)	Expert management for chronic GVHD and its complications available Appropriate resources for core specialties established (ophthalmology, dermatology, physiatry, psychology, and gynecology)	More emphasis on GVHD than on very late effects. Occasional patients early on after HSCT may relapse (leukemia relapses can happen even 3 y after HSCT) and be excluded from this clinic. Currently, many such models are separate for adults and pediatric survivors.
HSCT survivorship LTFU (usually ≥2 y after HSCT eligible)	Expert management for chronic GVHD and its complications available Excellent resources for early detection of very late complications (eg, coronary heart disease)	Logistically hard to establish, unless a large transplantation program

Adapted from Hashmi S, Carpenter P, Khera N, et al. Lost in transition: the essential need for long-term follow-up clinic for blood and marrow transplantation survivors. Biol Blood Marrow Transplant 2015;21(2):225-32; with permission.

ESSENTIALS OF HEMATOPOIETIC CELL TRANSPLANTATION

Some essential aspects of HCT that are helpful for clinicians caring for patients both before and after transplant are listed. This guide may be helpful for pediatricians, internists, primary care physicians, allied health practitioners (nurse practitioners, and physician assistants), hematologists, and oncologists.

1. When to refer to an HCT expert or a transplant center
   a. For high-risk hematologic malignancies: at diagnosis or after the first cycle of chemotherapy
   b. For severe aplastic anemia: at diagnosis
   c. For hemoglobinopathies: at diagnosis for thalassemia major for genetic diseases for which the only cure is HCT
   d. For high-risk neuroblastoma: at diagnosis or after the first cycle of chemotherapy
   e. For high-risk germ cell tumors: at diagnosis or after the first cycle of chemotherapy
2. How to manage GVHD
   a. Refer to the transplant center at diagnosis or suspicion of GVHD.
   b. Manage high-dose corticosteroid adverse effects, including high sugars, hypertension, insomnia, and so forth.
   c. Appropriate referral to specialist, for example, physical therapy for chronic GVHD contractures, ophthalmology for ocular GVHD, and so forth
3. Long-term survivorship issues
   a. Appropriate screening according to the ASBMT guidelines, for example, annual full dermatology screen for skin cancers, annual mammograms, thyroid-stimulating hormone checking per defined intervals, and so forth
   b. Screen for financial concerns and social distressors. Screen for posttraumatic stress disorder, depression, and anxiety

REFERENCES

1. Thomas ED, Lochte HL Jr, Lu WC, et al. Intravenous infusion of bone marrow in patients receiving radiation and chemotherapy. N Engl J Med 1957;257(11): 491–6.
2. Available at: https://bethematch.org/. Accessed December 1, 2015.
3. Gragert L, Eapen M, Williams E, et al. HLA match likelihoods for hematopoietic stem-cell grafts in the US registry. N Engl J Med 2014;371(4): 339–48.
4. Sorror ML, Maris MB, Storb R, et al. Hematopoietic Cell Transplantation (HCT)-specific comorbidity index: a new tool for risk assessment before allogeneic HCT. Blood 2005;106(8):2912–9.
5. Majhail NS, Farnia SH, Carpenter PA, et al. Indications for autologous and allogeneic hematopoietic cell transplantation: guidelines from the American Society for Blood and Marrow Transplantation. Biol Blood Marrow Transplant 2015;21(11): 1863–9.
6. Ferrara JL, Levine JE, Reddy P, et al. Graft-versus-host disease. Lancet 2009; 373(9674):1550–61.
7. Petersdorf EW, Malkki M, O'hUigin C, et al. High HLA-DP expression and graft-versus-host disease. N Engl J Med 2015;373(7):599–609.
8. Essig S, Li Q, Chen Y, et al. Risk of late effects of treatment in children newly diagnosed with standard-risk acute lymphoblastic leukaemia: a report from the Childhood Cancer Survivor Study cohort. Lancet Oncol 2014;15(8): 841–51.

9. Majhail NS, Rizzo JD, Lee SJ, et al. Recommended screening and preventive practices for long-term survivors after hematopoietic cell transplantation. Hematol oncol Stem Cell Ther 2012;5(1):1–30.

10. Hashmi S, Carpenter P, Khera N, et al. Lost in transition: the essential need for long-term follow-up clinic for blood and marrow transplantation survivors. Biol Blood Marrow Transplant 2015;21(2):225–32.

UNITED STATES POSTAL SERVICE®
Statement of Ownership, Management, and Circulation
(All Periodicals Publications Except Requester Publications)

1. Publication Title	2. Publication Number	3. Filing Date
PRIMARY CARE: CLINICS IN OFFICE PRACTICE	044 – 690	9/18/2016

4. Issue Frequency	5. Number of Issues Published Annually	6. Annual Subscription Price
MAR, JUN, SEP, DEC	4	$225.00

7. Complete Mailing Address of Known Office of Publication (Not printer) (Street, city, county, state, and ZIP+4®)

ELSEVIER INC.
360 PARK AVENUE SOUTH
NEW YORK, NY 10010-1710

Contact Person: STEPHEN R. BUSHING
Telephone (Include area code): 215-239-3688

8. Complete Mailing Address of Headquarters or General Business Office of Publisher (Not printer)

ELSEVIER INC.
360 PARK AVENUE SOUTH
NEW YORK, NY 10010-1710

9. Full Names and Complete Mailing Addresses of Publisher, Editor, and Managing Editor (Do not leave blank)

Publisher (Name and complete mailing address)

ADRIANNE BRIGIDO, ELSEVIER INC.
1600 JOHN F KENNEDY BLVD. SUITE 1800
PHILADELPHIA, PA 19103-2899

Editor (Name and complete mailing address)

JESSICA MCCOOL, ELSEVIER INC.
1600 JOHN F KENNEDY BLVD. SUITE 1800
PHILADELPHIA, PA 19103-2899

Managing Editor (Name and complete mailing address)

PATRICK MANLEY, ELSEVIER INC.
1600 JOHN F KENNEDY BLVD. SUITE 1800
PHILADELPHIA, PA 19103-2899

10. Owner (Do not leave blank. If the publication is owned by a corporation, give the name and address of the corporation immediately followed by the names and addresses of all stockholders owning or holding 1 percent or more of the total amount of stock. If not owned by a corporation, give the names and addresses of the individual owners. If owned by a partnership or other unincorporated firm, give its name and address as well as those of each individual owner. If the publication is published by a nonprofit organization, give its name and address.)

Full Name	Complete Mailing Address
WHOLLY OWNED SUBSIDIARY OF REED/ELSEVIER, US HOLDINGS	1600 JOHN F KENNEDY BLVD. SUITE 1800 PHILADELPHIA, PA 19103-2899

11. Known Bondholders, Mortgagees, and Other Security Holders Owning or Holding 1 Percent or More of Total Amount of Bonds, Mortgages, or Other Securities. If none, check box. ► ☐ None

Full Name	Complete Mailing Address
N/A	

12. Tax Status (For completion by nonprofit organizations authorized to mail at nonprofit rates) (Check one)
The purpose, function, and nonprofit status of this organization and the exempt status for federal income tax purposes:
☐ Has Not Changed During Preceding 12 Months
☐ Has Changed During Preceding 12 Months (Publisher must submit explanation of change with this statement)

PS Form 3526, July 2014 [Page 1 of 4 (see instructions page 4)] PSN: 7530-01-000-9931 PRIVACY NOTICE: See our privacy policy on www.usps.com.

13. Publication Title	14. Issue Date for Circulation Data Below
PRIMARY CARE: CLINICS IN OFFICE PRACTICE	JUNE 2016

15. Extent and Nature of Circulation		Average No. Copies Each Issue During Preceding 12 Months	No. Copies of Single Issue Published Nearest to Filing Date
a. Total Number of Copies (Net press run)		137	165
b. Paid Circulation (By Mail and Outside the Mail)	(1) Mailed Outside-County Paid Subscriptions Stated on PS Form 3541 (Include paid distribution above nominal rate, advertiser's proof copies, and exchange copies)	64	66
	(2) Mailed In-County Paid Subscriptions Stated on PS Form 3541 (Include paid distribution above nominal rate, advertiser's proof copies, and exchange copies)	0	0
	(3) Paid Distribution Outside the Mails Including Sales Through Dealers and Carriers, Street Vendors, Counter Sales, and Other Paid Distribution Outside USPS®	16	16
	(4) Paid Distribution by Other Classes of Mail Through the USPS (e.g. First-Class Mail®)	0	0
c. Total Paid Distribution [Sum of 15b (1), (2), (3), and (4)]	►	80	82
d. Free or Nominal Rate Distribution (By Mail and Outside the Mail)	(1) Free or Nominal Rate Outside-County Copies included on PS Form 3541	14	53
	(2) Free or Nominal Rate In-County Copies included on PS Form 3541	0	0
	(3) Free or Nominal Rate Copies Mailed at Other Classes Through the USPS (e.g. First-Class Mail)	0	0
	(4) Free or Nominal Rate Distribution Outside the Mail (Carriers or other means)	0	0
e. Total Free or Nominal Rate Distribution (Sum of 15d (1), (2), (3) and (4))	►	14	53
f. Total Distribution (Sum of 15c and 15e)	►	94	135
g. Copies not Distributed (See Instructions to Publishers #4 (page #3))	►	43	30
h. Total (Sum of 15f and g)	►	137	165
i. Percent Paid (15c divided by 15f times 100)		85%	59%

* If you are claiming electronic copies, go to line 16 on page 3. If you are not claiming electronic copies, skip to line 17 on page 3.

16. Electronic Copy Circulation		Average No. Copies Each Issue During Preceding 12 Months	No. Copies of Single Issue Published Nearest to Filing Date
a. Paid Electronic Copies	►	0	0
b. Total Paid Print Copies (Line 15c) + Paid Electronic Copies (Line 16a)	►	80	82
c. Total Print Distribution (Line 15f) + Paid Electronic Copies (Line 16a)	►	94	135
d. Percent Paid (Both Print & Electronic Copies) (16b divided by 16c × 100)	►	85%	59%

☒ I certify that 50% of all my distributed copies (electronic and print) are paid above a nominal price.

17. Publication of Statement of Ownership
☒ If the publication is a general publication, publication of this statement is required. Will be printed in the DECEMBER 2016 issue of this publication. ☐ Publication not required.

18. Signature and Title of Editor, Publisher, Business Manager, or Owner

STEPHEN R. BUSHING - INVENTORY DISTRIBUTION CONTROL MANAGER

Date: 9/18/2016

I certify that all information furnished on this form is true and complete. I understand that anyone who furnishes false or misleading information on this form or who omits material or information requested on the form may be subject to criminal sanctions (including fines and imprisonment) and/or civil sanctions (including civil penalties).

PS Form 3526, July 2014 (Page 3 of 4) PRIVACY NOTICE: See our privacy policy on www.usps.com.

Moving?

Make sure your subscription moves with you!

To notify us of your new address, find your **Clinics Account Number** (located on your mailing label above your name), and contact customer service at:

Email: journalscustomerservice-usa@elsevier.com

800-654-2452 (subscribers in the U.S. & Canada)
314-447-8871 (subscribers outside of the U.S. & Canada)

Fax number: 314-447-8029

Elsevier Health Sciences Division
Subscription Customer Service
3251 Riverport Lane
Maryland Heights, MO 63043

*To ensure uninterrupted delivery of your subscription, please notify us at least 4 weeks in advance of move.

Printed and bound by CPI Group (UK) Ltd, Croydon, CR0 4YY

07/10/2024

01040505-0012